Lessons Learned from Rhinologic Procedure Complications

Rakesh K. Chandra • Kevin C. Welch
Editors

Lessons Learned from Rhinologic Procedure Complications

A Case-Based Review

Springer

Editors
Rakesh K. Chandra
Otolaryngology-Head & Neck Surgery
Vanderbilt University Medical Center
Nashville, TN
USA

Kevin C. Welch
Otolaryngology-Head & Neck Surgery
Northwestern University/Northwestern
Medicine
Chicago, IL
USA

ISBN 978-3-030-75322-1 ISBN 978-3-030-75323-8 (eBook)
https://doi.org/10.1007/978-3-030-75323-8

This Springer imprint is published by the registered company Springer Nature Switzerland AG
The registered company address is: Gewerbestrasse 11, 6330 Cham, Switzerland

Foreword

There is always a need to review our poor results and complications in the surgery we perform. Of interest, when endoscopic sinus diagnosis and surgery was first introduced in the United States by Drs. Heinz Stammberger and David Kennedy in 1985, there was little discussion of complications. It was only until enthusiastic endoscopic sinus surgeons started performing the surgery that it became clear it was a potentially dangerous surgery. Indeed, historically, discussing ethmoid surgery in 1913, Dr. Mosher stated sinus surgery was hazardous and an easy way to kill a patient [1]. A number of serious eye and brain injury complications occurred early on which raised a red flag of caution to the sinus surgeons. Like any other new surgical procedure, an individual learning curve needed to be developed. The only training practitioners could get was in the early dissection courses; there was no residency training but more "on the job" training. Discussion about complication prevention and treatment became part of every endoscopic sinus surgery course and in residency training programs. With experience, anticipation, and preparation, the number of serious complication reduced but did not disappear. Also, it became apparent that experience even in my own case did not always excuse the surgeon from a complication even with the introduction of computerized guidance. The surgeon must always be vigilant and wary. Knowledge is the key based on preparation, anatomical and radiological objective data via endoscopy and CT scanning. Recognizing complications when they occur and initiating proper treatment in many cases can avoid permanent injury. I look forward to reading this unique case based book which will discuss how a complication occurred, review how that complication could have been avoided, and discussing what was learned through total case review and outcome. I hope it provides the reader with increased understanding and knowledge leading to greater patient safety.

Reference

1. Mosher HP. The applied anatomy and the intra-nasal surgery of the ethmoidal labyrinth. Laryngoscope. 1913;23:887–907.

James Stankiewicz, MD
Loyola University Medical Center,
Maywood, IL, USA

Contents

Contributors

Nithin D. Adappa, MD Department of Otorhinolaryngology - Head and Neck Surgery, University of Pennsylvania, Philadelphia, PA, USA

Jeremiah A. Alt, MD, PhD Division of Otolaryngology – Head and Neck Surgery, Rhinology-Sinus and Skull Base Surgery Program, Department of Surgery, University of Utah School of Medicine, Salt Lake City, UT, USA

Emily M. Barrow, MD Department of Otolaryngology, Head and Neck Surgery, Emory University School of Medicine, Atlanta, GA, USA

Daniel M. Beswick, MD Department of Head and Neck Surgery, University of California, Los Angeles, Los Angeles, CA, USA

Benjamin S. Bleier, MD, FACS, FARS Department of Otolaryngology, Massachusetts Eye and Ear Infirmary, Harvard Medical School, Boston, MA, USA

Taylor R. Carle, MD UCLA Department of Head and Neck Surgery, Los Angeles, CA, USA

Roy Casiano, MD Department of Otolaryngology, University of Miami, Miami, FL, USA

Mohamad R. Chaaban, MD, MSCR, MBA Head and Neck Institute, Cleveland Clinic, Cleveland, OH, USA

Rakesh K. Chandra, MD, MMHC, FACS Otolaryngology-Head & Neck Surgery, Vanderbilt University Medical Center, Nashville, TN, USA

Nikita Chapurin, MD, MHS Department of Otolaryngology – Head and Neck Surgery, Vanderbilt University Medical Center, Nashville, TN, USA

Alexander Chiu, MD Department of Otolaryngology-Head and Neck Surgery, University of Kansas Medical Center, Kansas City, KS, USA

Seth J. Davis, MD Department of Otolaryngology – Head & Neck Surgery, Vanderbilt University Medical Center, Nashville, TN, USA

Raj D. Dedhia, MD Department of Otolaryngology, University of Tennessee Health Science Center, Memphis, TN, USA

Division of Facial Plastic and Reconstructive Surgery, University of Tennessee Health Science Center, Memphis, TN, USA

John M. DelGaudio, MD Department of Otolaryngology, Head and Neck Surgery, Emory University School of Medicine, Atlanta, GA, USA

Sachi Dholakia, BS Department of Otolaryngology – Head and Neck Surgery, Stanford University School of Medicine, Stanford, CA, USA

Megan Falls, MD Indiana University School of Medicine, Indianapolis, IN, USA

Meha G. Fox, MD Department of Otolaryngology-Head and Neck Surgery, Baylor College of Medicine, Houston, TX, USA

Mark W. Gelpi, MD Division of Rhinology, Allergy, and Endoscopic Skull Base Surgery, University of North Carolina at Chapel Hill, Chapel Hill, NC, USA

Mathew N. Geltzeiler, MD University of Pittsburgh Medical Center, The Eye & Ear Institute, Pittsburgh, PA, USA

Amarbir S. Gill, MD Department of Otolaryngology – Head and Neck Surgery, University of California, Davis, Sacramento, CA, USA

Jessica W. Grayson, MD Department of Otolaryngology Head and Neck Surgery, University of Alabama Birmingham, Birmingham, AL, USA

David W. Kennedy, MD Department of Otorhinolaryngology – Head and Neck Surgery, University of Pennsylvania, Philadelphia, PA, USA

Dayoung Kim, BA Department of Otolaryngology – Head and Neck Surgery, Stanford University School of Medicine, Stanford, CA, USA

Kyle S. Kimura, MD Department of Otolaryngology – Head & Neck Surgery, Vanderbilt University Medical Center, Nashville, TN, USA

Todd T. Kingdom, MD Department of Otolaryngology – Head and Neck Surgery, University of Colorado, Aurora, CO, USA

Department of Ophthalmology, University of Colorado, Aurora, CO, USA

Devyani Lal, MD Mayo Clinic, Phoenix, AZ, USA

Ashton E. Lehmann, MD Department of Otolaryngology–Head and Neck Surgery, Vanderbilt University Medical Center, Nashville, TN, USA

Ryan E. Little, MD Department of Otolaryngology – Head and Neck Surgery, Medical University of South Carolina, Charleston, SC, USA

Tran B. Locke, MD Department of Otolaryngology – Head and Neck Surgery, Baylor College of Medicine, Houston, TX, USA

Michael J. Marino, MD Mayo Clinic, Phoenix, AZ, USA

Conner J. Massey, MD Department of Otolaryngology, University of Colorado School of Medicine, Aurora, CO, USA

William G. Morrel, MD Department of Otolaryngology – Head & Neck Surgery, Vanderbilt University Medical Center, Nashville, TN, USA

Jayakar V. Nayak, MD, PhD Department of Otolaryngology – Head and Neck Surgery, Stanford University School of Medicine, Stanford, CA, USA

James N. Palmer, MD Department of Otorhinolaryngology, Division of Rhinology, University of Pennsylvania Health System, Philadelphia, PA, USA

Katie Phillips, MD Department of Otolaryngology – Head and Neck Surgery, Stanford University School of Medicine, Stanford, CA, USA

Rodolfo Prestinary, MD Department of Otolaryngology, University of Miami, Miami, FL, USA

Vijay R. Ramakrishnan, MD Department of Otolaryngology, University of Colorado School of Medicine, Aurora, CO, USA

Rodney J. Schlosser, MD Department of Otolaryngology – Head and Neck Surgery, Medical University of South Carolina, Charleston, SC, USA

Brent A. Senior, MD, FACS, FARS Division of Rhinology, Allergy, and Endoscopic Skull Base Surgery, University of North Carolina at Chapel Hill, Chapel Hill, NC, USA

Raj Sindwani, MD Section of Rhinology, Sinus, and Skull Base Surgery, Head and Neck Institute, Cleveland Clinic, Cleveland, OH, USA

Minimally Invasive Cranial Base and Pituitary Surgery, Rosa Ella Burkhardt Brain Tumor & Neuro-Oncology Center, Cleveland Clinic, Cleveland, OH, USA

Toby O. Steele, MD Department of Otolaryngology – Head and Neck Surgery, University of California, Davis, Sacramento, CA, USA

Scott J. Stephan, MD Department of Otolaryngology – Head & Neck Surgery, Vanderbilt University Medical Center, Nashville, TN, USA

Division of Facial Plastic and Reconstructive Surgery, Vanderbilt University Medical Center, Nashville, TN, USA

Jeffrey D. Suh, MD UCLA Department of Head and Neck Surgery, Los Angeles, CA, USA

Dennis M. Tang, MD Department of Otolaryngology, Cedars-Sinai Medical Center, Los Angeles, CA, USA

Jonathan Ting, MD, MS, MBA Indiana University School of Medicine, Indianapolis, IN, USA

Charles C. L. Tong, MD Department of Otorhinolaryngology, Division of Rhinology, University of Pennsylvania Health System, Philadelphia, PA, USA

Jackson R. Vuncannon, MD Department of Otolaryngology, Head and Neck Surgery, Emory University School of Medicine, Atlanta, GA, USA

Eric W. Wang, MD University of Pittsburgh Medical Center, The Eye & Ear Institute, Pittsburgh, PA, USA

Kevin C. Welch, MD Otolaryngology-Head & Neck Surgery, Northwestern University/Northwestern Medicine, Chicago, IL, USA

Bradford A. Woodworth, MD, FACS Department of Otolaryngology Head and Neck Surgery, University of Alabama Birmingham, Birmingham, AL, USA

Angela Yang, BS Department of Otolaryngology – Head and Neck Surgery, Stanford University School of Medicine, Stanford, CA, USA

Part I
The Orbit

Chapter 1
Orbital Hematoma

Michael J. Marino and Devyani Lal

Clinical Pearls

1. The anterior and posterior ethmoidal arteries can get injured during endoscopic sinus surgery and result in a retro-orbital hematoma if they retract into the orbit.
2. Prompt recognition and management of an expanding retro-orbital hematoma can prevent visual change or loss.
3. The endoscopic sinus surgeon must be prepared to urgently manage an expanding retro-orbital hematoma by means of lateral canthotomy and cantholysis and/or orbital decompression.

Case Presentation

Patient presented to author MJM with a right ethmoid bony mass, which remodeled and displaced the medial orbital wall and anterior skull base. The patient noted right nasal congestion and frontal pain, although he denied changes in vision and diplopia. Sinus computed tomography (CT) and brain magnetic resonance imaging (MRI) were consistent with a bony mass, with the differential diagnosis including osteoma, fibrous dysplasia, and ossifying fibroma (Fig. 1.1). The patient elected for excisional biopsy of the mass by an endoscopic endonasal approach.

A 4 mm diamond burr was used to remove tumor from the medial orbital wall. While using the drill there was violation of the medial orbital wall in the area of the anterior ethmoid artery. Suspected orbital fat was seen to prolapse into the ethmoid cavity and drilling was immediately stopped (Fig. 1.2a). Bulb press maneuver by gentle compression on the external eye was performed and the presence of orbital

M. J. Marino · D. Lal (✉)
Mayo Clinic, Phoenix, AZ, USA
e-mail: lal.devyani@mayo.edu

R. K. Chandra, K. C. Welch (eds.), *Lessons Learned from Rhinologic Procedure Complications*, https://doi.org/10.1007/978-3-030-75323-8_1

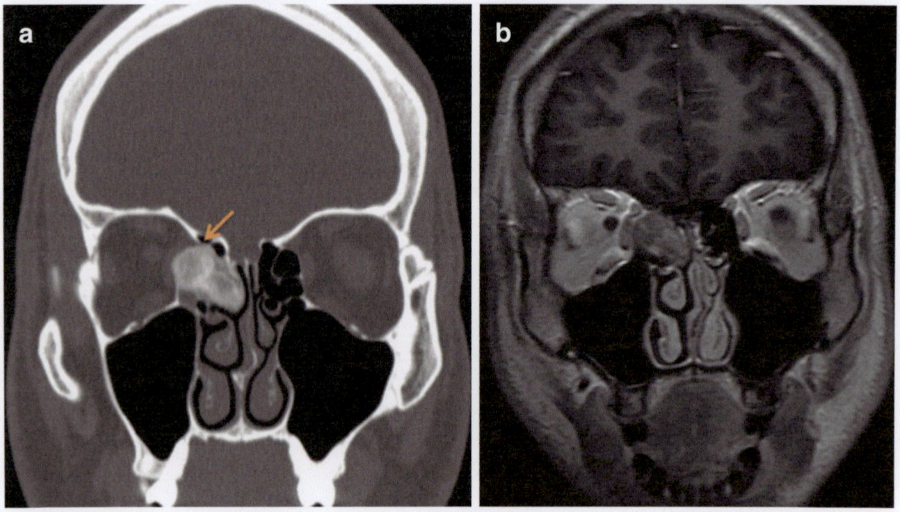

Fig. 1.1 Computed tomography (**a**) and magnetic resonance imaging (**b**) of ethmoid bony lesion along the orbit and skull base. Arrow designates the assumed location of the anterior ethmoid artery

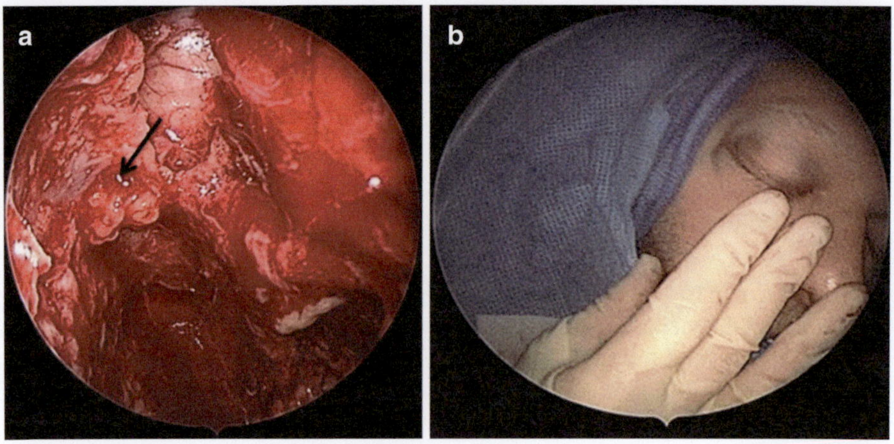

Fig. 1.2 Orbital fat is seen to prolapse into the ethmoid cavity (**a**). Ecchymosis and proptosis present after anterior ethmoid artery injury, heralding the development of an orbital hematoma (**b**)

fat and movement with compression in the surgical field was confirmed endoscopically. The external eye was noted to be soft to palpation during this initial bulb press maneuver. The anterior ethmoidal artery could not be visualized. Visual observation of the external eye over the next several minutes demonstrated rapid development of proptosis and periorbital ecchymosis (Fig. 1.2b). There was progressive firmness of the globe on palpation with bulb press maneuvers within minutes. The pupil was noted to be dilated and nonreactive to light.

The patient was immediately recognized to have developed an expanding orbital hematoma from anterior ethmoid artery injury. The anesthesia team was advised to administer intravenous mannitol (1 g/kg of 25% solution) and corticosteroids (10 mg dexamethasone). The ophthalmology team was consulted intraoperatively at the same time. The surgeon continued to gently massage the orbit and then proceeded with lateral canthotomy and cantholysis (Fig. 1.3). The globe was noted to immediately soften to palpation, and the pupil became reactive to light. Intraocular pressure was subsequently measured using a tonometer in conjunction with the ophthalmologist, and was found to be 18 mm Hg.

The case was aborted after orbital decompression, and the patient was awakened, extubated, and transferred to the post-anesthesia care unit. Visual acuity and extraocular muscle function was tested in the post-anesthesia care unit, and found to be within normal limits. The patient was observed overnight to ensure no further development of hematoma, or changes in visual acuity and extraocular muscle function. He was discharged home on postoperative day #1 without changes in vision or

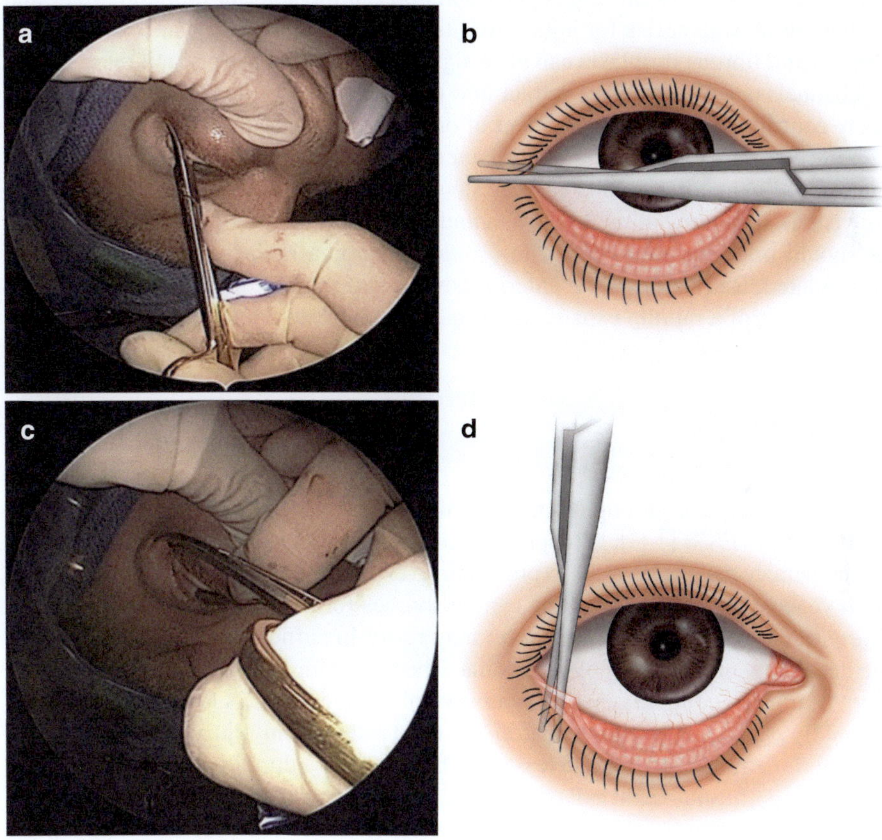

Fig. 1.3 Lateral canthotomy is performed by using sharp scissors to incise from the lateral commissure to the orbital rim (**a**). Illustration of the lateral canthotomy procedure (**b**). Lateral cantholysis is then performed by directing the scissors inferiorly to cut the lateral canthal tendon (**c**). Illustration of the lateral cantholysis procedure (**d**)

diplopia. At 6 month follow-up the patient had complete healing of the lateral canthotomy and cantholysis incisions without aesthetic change.

Root Cause Analysis

Several factors contributed to orbital hematoma complication in this case. First, surgical anatomy was distorted by the lesion, and particularly common surgical landmarks. Loss of anatomical landmarks contributed to a second difficulty in accurately determining the location of the anterior ethmoid artery. Computerized image guidance was utilized during surgery, but this technology does not replace endoscopic visualization and identification of critical structures. Use of image guidance may not necessarily prevent complications. Furthermore, instrumentation used for removing the bony lesion (high-speed burr) placed the anterior ethmoid artery and medial orbital wall at risk for injury. Additionally, bony pathology such as ossifying fibroma and fibrous dysplasia can have significant vascular supply and these vascular channels can also bleed or retract into the orbit. The confluence of these factors likely contributed to the development of orbital hematoma.

Arterial injury was likely a major factor in the development of clinically significant orbital hematoma in this case. A slow hematoma may develop from injury to the venous structures in the periorbita and orbital fat, although exposure of orbital fat should not necessarily result in orbital hematoma if the area of injury is not manipulated. Retraction of the anterior ethmoid artery into the orbit resulted in the development of a rapidly expanding retro-orbital hematoma in this case.

Lessons Learned

Orbital hematoma is among the most common major complications of endoscopic sinus surgery (ESS) [1–3]. Prompt recognition and treatment of an expanding retro-orbital hematoma is necessary to prevent irreversible changes in visual acuity [1, 2]. Both venous and arterial bleeding can be sources for orbital hematoma formation. Injury to the periorbita and orbital fat may result in sufficient venous bleeding for the development of an orbital hematoma. The time course of a hematoma resulting from venous bleeding may range from several minutes to days following the event. A rapidly expanding orbital hematoma is most likely from injury and retraction of the anterior ethmoid artery, and less often the posterior ethmoid artery. Tumors such as ossifying fibroma, renal cell carcinoma, or any vascular tumor can also bleed into the orbit during tumor resection, and the surgeon should be prepared with a plan. The eye should be always left exposed while draping for endoscopic sinus surgery. The surgical team should be briefed to the high risk of orbital complications in these cases so that surgical instrumentation such as angled endoscopic bipolar cautery can be quickly available. Availability of a sharp cutting pair of scissors should be assured prior to dissection.

The anterior ethmoid and, less commonly, the posterior artery can lie in the ethmoid cavity on a mesentery or be dehiscent in their canals. Hyper-pneumatized ethmoid air cells are particularly associated with pedicled ethmoidal arteries, which then become especially vulnerable to injury during ESS if not recognized on preoperative CT scan and avoided during surgical dissection. If the artery is transected close to the lateral end the vessel may retract into the orbit. Rapid orbital hematoma formation and expansion can result in blindness within 30 minutes from an arterial source and within 90 minutes from a venous source, demanding prompt identification and management in order to avoid irreversible visual changes [1].

Clinical signs of orbital hematoma can vary, and should be vigilantly monitored in the setting of a known lamina papyracea, orbital fat, and arterial injury during ESS and during any nasal tumor surgery. Initial findings may be limited to periorbital ecchymosis and lid edema, with progression to chemosis, proptosis, afferent pupillary defect, and dilated and nonreactive pupil. Firmness of the globe to palpation is an additional sign of developing orbital hematoma, and preoperative palpation is essential for appreciation of intraoperative changes. The pupillary reaction and the firmness of the orbit should be carefully monitored and be the guide to urgency of action. Use of transparent or non-occlusive eye taping during ESS is recommended so that the surgeon can recognize these signs, particularly in the setting of a suspected injury. In the case presented in this chapter, there was rapid progression of periorbital ecchymosis and proptosis, as well as a firm globe on palpation, prompting management for orbital hematoma.

Upon suspicion of an orbital hematoma the operating team should be clearly informed of the plan of action. Ophthalmology consult should be obtained urgently. Familiarity with a tonometer is also recommended and the operating team can measure intraocular pressure (IOP) prior to the availability of ophthalmology consult. Ideally, the location of a tonometer should be known to the surgical team. IOP above 30 mmHg may result in vision compromise [2], and management steps for orbital hematoma should be started. Nevertheless, urgent management of the orbit should not await availability of the tonometer or an ophthalmologist. Orbital massage can be initiated to redistribute orbital blood and fluids, and may reduce IOP. Medical management including intravenous mannitol (1 g/kg of 15–25% solution over 30 minutes) and dexamethasone (10 mg for adult patients) can be simultaneously started by the anesthesia team. Removal of any nasal packing and elevation of the head of bed may also be helpful for reducing IOP. Immediate consideration should then be given to lateral canthotomy and cantholysis when IOP remains elevated despite these initial measures.

Lateral canthotomy and cantholysis can be performed quickly during ESS or at the bedside in the postoperative setting. Canthotomy can result in a 15 mmHg decrease in IOP, while cantholysis can achieve an additional 20 mmHg decrease in IOP [4, 5]. The canthotomy procedure is performed by cutting from the lateral commissure to the orbital rim using sharp scissors (Fig. 1.3a, c). The scissors are then directed inferiorly and superiorly to cut the lateral canthal tendon in order to perform lateral cantholysis (Fig. 1.3b, d). The canthal tendon can often be palpated digitally or with the scissors, guiding the incision for cantholysis. The technique for both lateral canthotomy and cantholysis can be practiced and mastered on a cadaver specimen. Ability to perform these procedures should be essential for the endoscopic sinus surgeon in order to prevent irreversible vision change from orbital hematoma. After lateral canthotomy and cantholysis there is typically softening of the globe and reductions in IOP can be measured using a tonometer. In the presented case IOP dropped to 18 mmHg following these procedures, indicating that increased pressure within the orbit from the evolving hematoma had been successfully managed. In the event that the globe remains firm or IOP continues to be elevated after lateral canthotomy and cantholysis, consideration should be given at that point to proceeding with medial orbital decompression. Lateral canthotomy and cantholysis may be chosen over endoscopic medial orbital decompression for several reasons. The presence of the tumor made medial orbital decompression unviable in this case. Lateral canthotomy and cantholysis is also a quicker procedure. Finally, in patients undergoing ESS for CRS, orbital decompression may impact drainage of the sphenoid and frontal sinuses.

Medial orbital decompression may be indicated in rare situations where IOP does not improve despite lateral canthotomy. In a large series examining complications of ESS, including 20 orbital hematomas, progression to medial orbital decompression was only necessary in one case [1]. Medial orbital decompression can be performed endoscopically by removing the lamina papyracea (Fig. 1.4). Complete anterior and posterior ethmoidectomy should be performed in order to completely visualize the lamina papyracea and remove all attached ethmoid partitions. The lamina paprycea can then be carefully fractured and elevated from the underlying periorbita using a Freer elevator. The periorbita is then incised using a sickle knife in a direction parallel to the medial rectus muscle, thereby reducing the risk of injury to this critical structure. The globe is then gently massaged with prolapse of orbital fat into the surgical ethmoid cavity. If the source of arterial bleeding from the anterior or posterior ethmoid artery can be identified, this can be controlled with bipolar cautery. Monopolar cautery should be avoided since this can result in injury to important orbital and skull base structures, and potentially cause cerebrospinal fluid leak.

Postoperative management should include avoiding the use of nasal packing, which may adversely impact orbital decompression. Ophthalmology consult should be completed and document visual acuity and extraocular motion. The patient and the family should be informed of the injury. In the event that medial orbital decompression is necessary for management of increased IOP, postoperative diplopia may be present due to changes in globe position. Inpatient observation is recommended in the immediate postoperative period in order to ensure there is no further hemorrhage and hematoma formation, and to confirm there are no changes in visual acuity or extraocular motion. The plan for treatment and monitoring should be shared with the patient and observing team so that the surgeon can be immediately informed of any worrisome symptoms. In situations where lateral canthotomy and cantholysis was performed, canthopexy can be considered following resolution of the acute

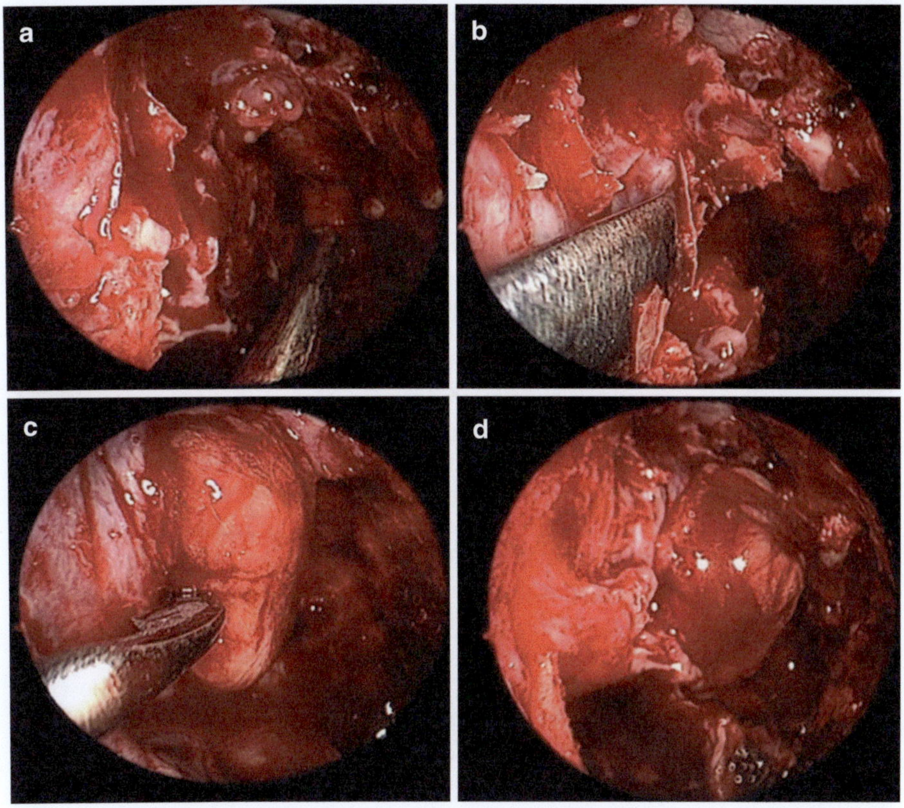

Fig. 1.4 The lamina papyracea is identified with endoscopic visualization (**a**), and then fractured and elevated from the periorbital using a Freer elevator (**b**). The periorbital is then incised in a posterior to anterior direction parallel to the medial rectus muscle (**c**), and orbital fat is exposed and massaged into the surgical field (**d**)

complication for cosmetic deformities. Aesthetic results following lateral canthotomy and cantholysis are generally well accepted by most patients.

Several considerations are also important for the prevention of orbital complications. The sinus CT should be carefully examined preoperatively and scrutinized for features that may increase the risk of orbital injury. Areas of dehiscence in the lamina papyracea should be noted, and history of prior ESS may be a contributing factor. The disease subtype should also be considered when reviewing preoperative imaging. For example, patients with allergic fungal rhinosinusitis commonly have thinning of bony structures resulting in dehiscence of the lamina papyracea. Tumors may distort the normal surgical anatomy, as in the case presented in this chapter, and a vascular tumor can also potentially bleed into the orbit once the periorbita is violated. Selection of procedures in pathology with significant anatomical distortion should be carefully evaluated. Furthermore, vascular structures may be vulnerable to injury due to normal anatomic variation in the paranasal sinuses. The degree of pneumatization of the supraorbital ethmoid cell is a landmark for identifying dehiscent anterior ethmoid artery that can be injured during surgery [6].

Imaging should always be available for review intraoperatively during ESS, as this can aid the surgeon in the event anatomy becomes distorted during the case. Consideration should also be given for image-guided surgery (IGS), particularly in situations of revision surgery, complex anatomy, frontal and sphenoid sinusotomy, nasal polyps, and sinonasal tumors. A meta-analysis demonstrated a decreased risk of total and major complications when IGS was used during ESS, although there was not a decreased risk of orbital complications specifically [7]. IGS was used during the case presented, and illustrates that computer navigation does not replace anatomic knowledge and endoscopic visualization. Nevertheless, IGS was still useful in this situation in helping to identify the area of injury and raise suspicion that the anterior ethmoid artery had been injured.

Additional intraoperative considerations can aid in preventing or promptly recognizing orbital complications. Powered instrumentation can create risks for orbital injury. Therefore, powered microdebriders should be completely visualized when being used, and the cutting blade should be directed away from or parallel to the orbit. Similar visualization should always be maintained when using drills, and non-powered instruments can be considered when removing bone from vascular structures. In the presented case, a high-speed burr was involved in injury to the anterior ethmoid artery, and dissection using non-powered instruments in this critical location may have been useful for preventing the injury. More generally, if endoscopic visualization is compromised the procedure should be stopped until hemostasis can be achieved, and potentially aborted if effective hemostasis is not possible.

Orbital hematoma is a potential major complication of ESS and can threaten vision. Prompt recognition of this complication and the potential causes is essential for managing the situation and preventing long-term morbidity. Lateral canthotomy and cantholysis are effective at decreasing IOP and can be performed quickly during ESS or at the bedside postoperatively. These procedures can be easily mastered with practice using cadaver specimens, and are essential tools for the endoscopic sinus surgeon. Prevention and preparation are also important factors for avoiding morbidity due to orbital hematoma. Careful preoperative review of imaging and pathology is useful for both preventing orbital injury and maximizing preparation in the event that a complication occurs. Technological resources such as IGS, while not protective against complications, may be helpful in identifying anatomical structures during a complication. Overall, orbital hematoma can be managed successfully with meticulous preoperative planning, intraoperative awareness and familiarity with important treatment interventions.

References

1. Stankiewicz JA, Lal D, Connor M, Welch K. Complications in endoscopic sinus surgery for chronic rhinosinusitis: a 25-year experience. Laryngoscope. 2011;121(12):2684–701.

2. Patel AB, Hoxworth JM, Lal D. Orbital complications associated with the treatment of chronic rhinosinusitis. Otolaryngol Clin N Am. 2015;48(5):749–68.
3. Ramakrishnan VR, Kingdom TT, Nayak JV, Hwang PH, Orlandi RR. Nationwide incidence of major complications in endoscopic sinus surgery. Int Forum Allergy Rhinol. 2012;2(1):34–9.
4. Ramakrishnan VR, Palmer JN. Prevention and management of orbital hematoma. Otolaryngol Clin N Am. 2010;43(4):789–800.
5. Yung CW, Moorthy RS, Lindley D, Ringle M, Nunery WR. Efficacy of lateral canthotomy and cantholysis in orbital hemorrhage. Ophthalmic Plast Reconstr Surg. 1994;10(2):137–41.
6. Jang DW, Lachanas VA, White LC, Kountakis SE. Supraorbital ethmoid cell: a consistent landmark for endoscopic identification of the anterior ethmoidal artery. Otolaryngol Head Neck Surg. 2014;151(6):1073–7.
7. Dalgorf DM, Sacks R, Wormald PJ, et al. Image-guided surgery influences perioperative morbidity from endoscopic sinus surgery: a systematic review and meta-analysis. Otolaryngol Head Neck Surg. 2013;149(1):17–29.

Chapter 2
Management of Orbital Hematoma in Endoscopic Sinus Surgery

Charles C. L. Tong and James N. Palmer

Clinical Pearls

1. Injury to the anterior ethmoid artery during sinus surgery is a rare complication that can lead to orbital hematoma. Successful management requires the surgeon to be aptly trained in recognition, cauterization, and orbital decompression techniques.
2. Careful evaluation of the preoperative imaging can often identify the location of the anterior ethmoidal canal. The artery is most prone to injury during ethmoid sinus dissection, and the anterior ethmoid canal is found to be below the skull base in about 15% of the general population.
3. In the event of an orbital compartment syndrome, the surgeon must be decisive with medical and surgical interventions. Rapid decompression of the orbit can be achieved with a lateral canthotomy and cantholysis.

Case Presentation

A 27-year-old female referred to tertiary rhinology practice 2 weeks after surgery for presumed inflammatory disease. Pathology revealed poorly differentiated squamous cell carcinoma and patient presents for definitive treatment. Her nasal endoscopy revealed significant sinonasal edema and no clear tumor pedicle was identified. She had no other pertinent past medical or surgical history. Of note, she denied any visual disturbances or history of facial trauma. Coronal images of her preoperative CT and post-contrast MRI can be seen in Fig. 2.1. The patient was counseled on the

C. C. L. Tong · J. N. Palmer (✉)
Department of Otorhinolaryngology, Division of Rhinology, University of Pennsylvania Health System, Philadelphia, PA, USA
e-mail: james.palmer@uphs.upenn.edu

R. K. Chandra, K. C. Welch (eds.), *Lessons Learned from Rhinologic Procedure Complications*, https://doi.org/10.1007/978-3-030-75323-8_2

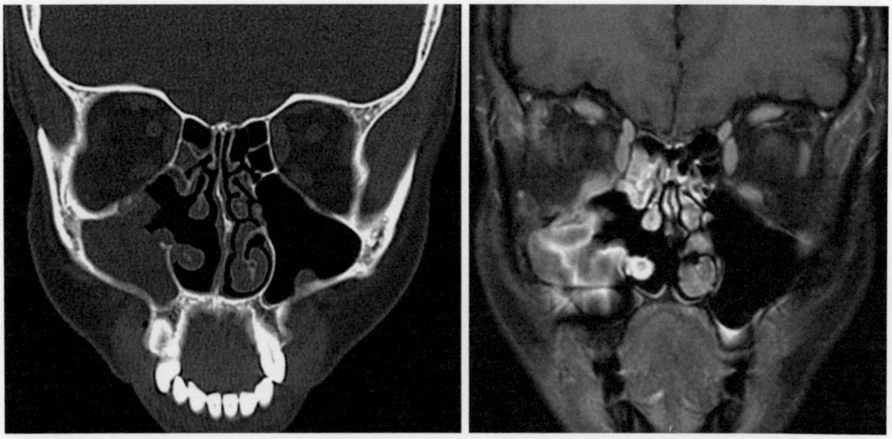

Fig. 2.1 *Left:* Coronal CT image of a patient with tissue-biopsy-proven malignancy showing partially dissected sinus cavities. *Right:* A T1-weighted post-contrast MRI image reveals only polypoid inflammatory mucosal thickening without gross evidence of contrast enhancing lesion

significance of the pathology and decided to proceed with definitive surgery to appropriately map the tumor and for possible complete extirpation. She was properly informed of the risks of endoscopic sinus surgery, including the risks of CSF leak, orbital injury with temporary or permanent vision loss, nasal bleeding, epiphora, loss of smell, and the potential for additional future procedures.

Intraoperatively, there was diseased tissue along the posterior wall of the maxillary sinus and onto the lamina papyracea. These areas were removed. Residual ethmoid partitions were then dissected, and during this dissection, the right anterior ethmoid artery was injured (Fig. 2.2a). Shortly after the injury, orbital proptosis was recognized by visualization and palpation of the orbit. A tonometer was used to obtain the intraocular pressure (IOP): the left eye (uninjured eye) had a pressure of 18 mm Hg, while the IOP of the right eye (proptotic eye) had a pressure of 25 mm Hg. Ligation of the distal end of the right anterior ethmoid artery was achieved using the Dessi bipolar electrocautery (Fig. 2.2b). Orbital decompression was then performed in less than 5 minutes, exposing the proximal end of the AEA for cauterization. First, the entire lamina papyracea was taken down from the maxillary sinus roof up to the skull base, and anteriorly to the lacrimal duct and posteriorly to the orbital apex (Fig. 2.2c). This exposed the periobita, which was then incised using a sickle knife (Fig. 2.2d). The orbit was then decompressed with orbital fat herniating into the nasal cavity. Repeat tonometry found both eye pressures to be at 18 mm Hg. The rest of the procedure was completed uneventfully. Postoperatively, an ophthalmology consult was performed and confirmed baseline visual acuity. There was no defect in the visual fields. There was some periorbital swelling and bruising, evident in the immediate postoperative photograph, which resolved by POD7 (Fig. 2.3).

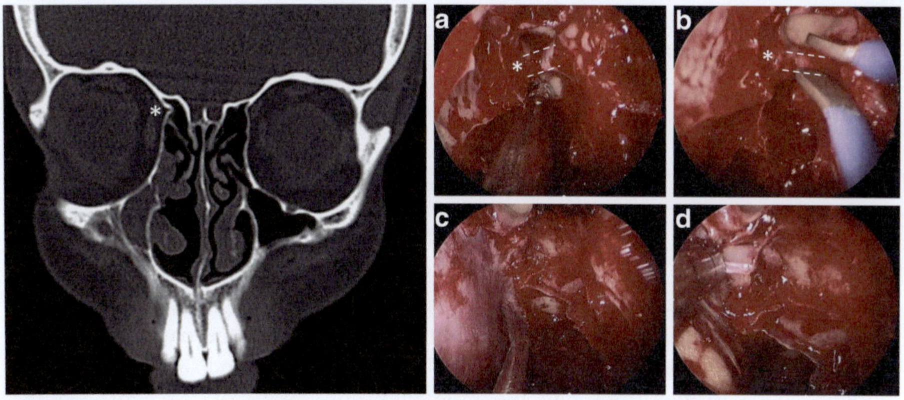

Fig. 2.2 *Left:* Review of coronal CT imaging reveals that the right anterior ethmoid artery is below the skull base. *Right:* The asterisk denotes the proximal course of the anterior ethmoid artery. (**a**) The bleeding vessel was identified and confirmed with image guidance. (**b**) A Dessi bipolar was used to cauterize the vessel. (**c**) The lamina papyracea was dissected off exposing the periorbita. A sickle knife was used to incise the periorbita. (**d**) The orbit is decompressed, periorbital fat is exposed

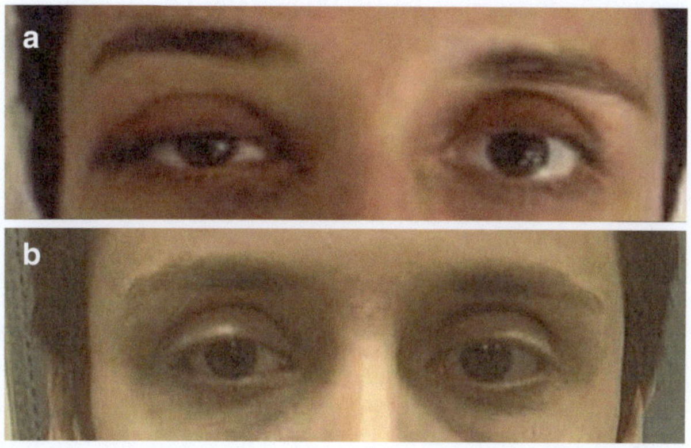

Fig. 2.3 (**a**) Immediate postoperative photograph. Some ecchymoses and periorbital swelling of the right orbit. Ocular testing was otherwise normal. (**b**) POD7 photograph. Orbital complications grossly resolved

Root Cause Analysis

In our case, the injury to the anterior ethmoid artery was recognized intraoperatively. Electrocautery was attempted with the Dessi bipolar forceps but the proximal end retracted into the orbit. Several factors contributed to the AEA injury and subsequent orbital hematoma. The pathology of the patient's disease dictated an aggressive approach with complete resection if possible. Unfortunately, there was diseased tissue along the entire medial wall of the orbit with extension to the ethmoid skull base. Combined with a dehiscent artery, the risk of injury was much higher than other routine endoscopic procedures. Furthermore, while the injury was recognized immediately, the proximal end of the vessel had retracted and intranasal bipolar electrocautery was insufficient in ligating the artery. The artery was eventually exposed and cauterized, with the medial wall taken down and the orbit appropriately decompressed. If presented with a similar case in the future, we would consider preemptively ligating the artery before proceeding with the dissection.

Lessons Learned

Over the past three decades, endoscopic sinus surgery has been widely recognized as a safe and efficacious treatment modality for diseases of the paranasal sinuses and anterior skull base. Advances in surgical instrumentation and stereotactic image guidance have further improved the efficiency and safety of these procedures. Despite the constant technological updates and innovation, complications can still arise and must be properly managed.

Among the most dreaded risks encountered in endoscopic sinus surgery is excessive bleeding from the anterior ethmoid artery into the orbit, which unrecognized, will result in the rapid formation of an orbital hematoma. This, in turn, will greatly increase the intraocular pressure, compromising the retinal blood supply and resulting in blindness in as few as 90 minutes [1, 2]. Fortunately, this complication is rare and its incidence can be mitigated by thorough preoperative planning and a stepwise management approach.

Anatomy of the Orbit and the Anterior Ethmoid Artery

The orbit is comprised of seven bones: frontal, zygoma, maxilla, lacrimal, ethmoid, palatine, and sphenoid. These bones form a bony pyramid that contains the globe, orbital fat, extraocular muscles, and neurovascular structures. It measures approximately 4 cm wide by 3.5 cm high at the base (orbital entrance), and 5 cm long to the apex of the orbital pyramid [3]. The orbits are slightly rotated laterally, with the thickness of the orbital walls varying but generally thinnest along the medial aspect. The overall orbital volume is approximately 30 mL, of which only 7 mL is occupied by the globe [4].

The medial wall is most often known as the lamina papyracea, which is roughly rectangular and extends from the frontal process of the maxilla to the orbital apex. This paper-thin bone is prone to fractures due to blunt maxillofacial trauma; therefore, its contour and thickness must be carefully reviewed prior to ethmoid sinus surgery. Preoperative defects of the lamina papyracea can best be identified on coronal and axial planes of thin sliced CT images (1.0–3.0 mm).

At the apex of the orbit is the optic canal, which permits passage of the optic nerve and ophthalmic artery, from which arise the anterior and posterior ethmoid arteries. These vessels perforate the nasal cavity through the frontoethmoidal suture and travel in grooves along the surface of the horizontal portion of the ethmoid bone.

The anterior ethmoid artery is a critical structure to identify when clearing the skull base and opening the frontal recess. To examine these relationships, a group of investigators performed an extensive dissection of 70 cadaveric heads and found the anterior ethmoidal canal to be located between the second and third lamella in 61 out of 70 cases [5]. This corresponds to the area between the ethmoid bulla and the basal lamella of the middle turbinate. They also found that the mean distance and angle between the limen nasi and the anterior ethmoidal canal were 4.9 cm and 54.5°, respectively. In 10 out of 70 cases (14.3%), the anterior ethmoidal canals were below the skull base at 2–3 mm, which would be most prone to injury to the unsuspecting surgeon. With close inspection of preoperative sagittal CT images, the anterior ethmoidal canal can be found within a bony swelling of the skull base between the second and third lamella. Coronal CT images can further aid identification by a bony "nipple" at the confluence of the medial rectus and superior oblique muscles indicating the nasal origin of the anterior ethmoid artery (Fig. 2.2). This bony structure can be seen on preoperative CT images to help identify a potential source of significant bleeding during complete dissection along the skull base. Moreover, through using stereotactic image-guided surgery, this landmark can be continually assessed intraoperatively during dissection to help avoid bleeding complications.

Intraoperative Management of Anterior Ethmoid Artery Injury

Prevention of intraoperative bleeding begins with an appropriate preoperative history and physical examination, with appropriate attention to the patient's medical history, bleeding history, use of antiplatelet or anticoagulation therapy, user of over-the-counter herbal or alternative medicine, hematocrit, hemoglobin, platelet count, and coagulation factors status (i.e., prothrombin time, international normalized ratio, and partial thromboplastin time). If the benefits outweigh its risk, pharmacological anticoagulation therapy should be halted and its duration be discussed with the patient's internist.

Preparation of the nasal cavity before surgery is essential. The nasal mucosa should be decongested with pledges moistened with oxymetazoline, phenylephrine, or cocaine solution for at least 10 minutes prior to performing endoscopic surgery. Transnasal or transoral injection of 1% lidocaine with 1:100,000 epinephrine to address the sphenopalatine artery can be considered. In conjunction with total intravenous anesthesia, permissive hypotension, relative bradycardia, these efforts can help minimize intraoperative blood loss while optimizing visualization and thus preventing intraoperative complications.

A complement of electrocautery devices, topical decongestants, and thrombin-activated hemostatic matrix should be readily available to the surgeon so that potential intraoperative bleeding may be addressed readily. The authors routinely have the following equipment and supplies available: monopolar suction cautery, Dessi bipolar forceps, 1:1000 epinephrine pledgets, thrombin-soaked pledgets, thrombin-infused gelatin or collagen matrix.

When an orbital hematoma is recognized, it constitutes an ophthalmologic emergency. The most common cause for the sinus surgeon is an arterial injury to the anterior ethmoid artery, and bleeding into the orbit can result in an orbital compartment syndrome with permanent injury to the optic nerve if ischemia time reaches 90–120 minutes [1, 2]. In our case, the injury to the anterior ethmoid artery was recognized intraoperatively. Electrocautery was attempted with the Dessi bipolar forceps but the proximal end retracted into the orbit. While the orbit may not be grossly proptotic initially, palpation and subsequent IOP measurement help confirm the suspected hematoma. Early signs of an orbital hematoma include preseptal edema, ecchymosis, orbital proptosis, and raised intraocular pressures (normal range, 10–20 mm Hg). Intraocular pressure can be determined by a tonometer (Fig. 2.4a, b). If the IOP is elevated, massage of the eye, administration of mannitol at 1–2 g/kg over 30 minutes as a 15–25% solution, and administration of 10 mg of intravenous dexamethasone are indicated. In the awake patient, timolol 0.5%, at 1–2 drops twice daily can help reduce IOP through decreased production of aqueous humor. These conservative measures may fail to reduce IOP acutely, and in our patient, we performed an orbital decompression with cauterization of the proximal stump of the anterior ethmoid artery. Immediate canthotomy and cantholysis must

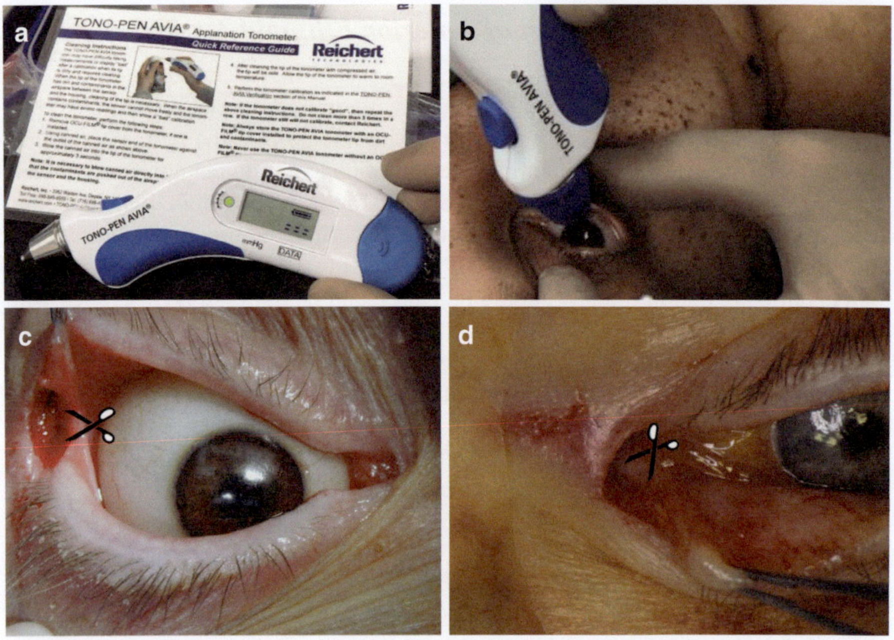

Fig. 2.4 (**a**) Handheld tonometer to measure intraocular pressure. (**b**) Measurement of IOP by gentle repeated tapping of the cornea. (**c**) Steps for performing a lateral canthotomy and cantholysis. The lateral canthus is incised beginning at the lateral lid commissure down to the lateral orbital rim. (**d**) The inferior crus of the lateral canthal tendon is then divided by pointing the curved Iris scissors inferiorly

be considered if the IOP is greater than 40 mm Hg, Marcus-Gunn pupil (defective afferent pupillary pathway), cherry red macula (central retinal artery occlusion), and severe retro-orbital pain if the patient is awake.

To perform a lateral canthotomy, 1% lidocaine with 1:100,000 epinephrine is administered to the lateral canthus. A hemostat may be used to crimp the skin of the lateral canthus to further assist with hemostasis. Next, a curved Iris scissors is used to incise the lateral commissure down to the periosteum of the lateral orbital rim. To perform the cantholysis, the inferior lateral canthal tendon must be released by cutting down inferiorly while retracting the lower lid (Fig. 2.4c, d). The sequential procedures of canthotomy and cantholysis have been shown to reduce the IOP by nearly 40% [6]. The repair can then be performed when IOP returns to normal and the source of bleeding controlled. Postoperatively, an ophthalmology consult is often encouraged to serially measure IOP, document visual acuity, and plan for further treatment.

Summary

Intraoperative orbital hematoma constitutes an emergency, and proper management is paramount in preserving vision. Thorough preoperative planning and careful dissection help mitigate the risk for anterior ethmoid artery injury; however, if an injury occurs, a stepwise approach and timely administration of intravenous medications and appropriate use of canthotomy with or without cantholysis can reduce complications related to orbital compartment syndrome. Consultation with an ophthalmologist is encouraged for serial visual acuity examination and continuity of care.

References

1. Popat H, Doyle PT, Davies SJ. Blindness following retrobulbar haemorrhage–it can be prevented. Br J Oral Maxillofac Surg. 2007;45:163–4. https://doi.org/10.1016/j.bjoms.2005.06.028.
2. Larsen M, Wieslander S. Acute orbital compartment syndrome after lateral blow-out fracture effectively relieved by lateral cantholysis. Acta Ophthalmol Scand. 1999;77:232–3. https://doi.org/10.1034/j.1600-0420.1999.770225.x.
3. Rootman J. Orbital surgery: a conceptual approach. 2nd ed. Lippincott Williams and Wilkins; 2013. ISBN: 978-1451100105.
4. Kikkawa D, Lemke B. In: Dortzbach RK, editor. Ophthalmic plastic surgery: prevention and management of complications. Lippincott Williams and Wilkins; 1994. p. 1–29. ISBN: 978-0781700290.
5. Moon HJ, Kim HU, Lee JG, Chung IH, Yoon JH. Surgical anatomy of the anterior ethmoidal canal in ethmoid roof. Laryngoscope. 2001;111:900–4. https://doi.org/10.1097/00005537-200105000-00027.
6. Mohammadi F, et al. Intraocular pressure changes in emergent surgical decompression of orbital compartment syndrome. JAMA Otolaryngol Head Neck Surg. 2015;141:562–5. https://doi.org/10.1001/jamaoto.2015.0524.

Chapter 3
Extraocular Muscle Injury

Brent A. Senior and Mark W. Gelpi

Clinical Pearls

1. Understand the relationships of the medial orbital wall and anterior ethmoid artery foramen with respect to the extraocular muscles. Anteriorly, the muscles are protected by a larger cushion of fat whereas posteriorly they are in intimate association with the medial orbital wall, allowing little room for error.
2. Utilize a preoperative checklist to identify pertinent patient-specific anatomy. This allows the surgeon to create a mental roadmap for sinus cavity dissection and avoid potential pitfalls.
3. Utilize meticulous dissection technique, with the force of dissection being parallel to the medial orbital wall. The microdebrider should be used cautiously and sparingly along the medial orbital wall.

Case Presentation

A 63 year-old otherwise healthy male presented with chief complaints of long-standing nasal obstruction, rhinorrhea, facial pressure, and loss of sense of smell. He had previously been treated by his primary care physician with multiple rounds of antibiotics, intranasal corticosteroids, and oral steroids without improvement.

B. A. Senior (✉) · M. W. Gelpi
Division of Rhinology, Allergy, and Endoscopic Skull Base Surgery, University of North Carolina at Chapel Hill, Chapel Hill, NC, USA
e-mail: Brent_Senior@med.unc.edu

R. K. Chandra, K. C. Welch (eds.), *Lessons Learned from Rhinologic Procedure Complications*, https://doi.org/10.1007/978-3-030-75323-8_3

Rigid nasal endoscopy revealed extensive nasal polyposis and mucopurulence bilaterally. A preoperative CT revealed diffuse polyposis filling the bilateral sinonasal cavities with near-total opacification of the sinuses. After discussion regarding ongoing medical versus surgical treatment options, the decision was made to proceed with surgery. The patient was taken to the operating room where bilateral functional endoscopic sinus surgery (FESS) was performed. Both powered instrumentation and image guidance were utilized through the entirety of the case. The case was notable for above-average bleeding during polypectomy obscuring normal landmarks as well as some uncharacteristic-looking polyps and heavy bleeding encountered during the left-sided maxillary antrostomy and ethmoidectomy. After the case, while in the post-anesthesia care unit, the patient complained of diplopia. Further examination revealed periorbital ecchymosis, left eye chemosis, and subconjunctival hemorrhage. There was limited depression and adduction of the right globe as well as slight lateralization of the globe with straight-ahead gaze (Fig. 3.1).

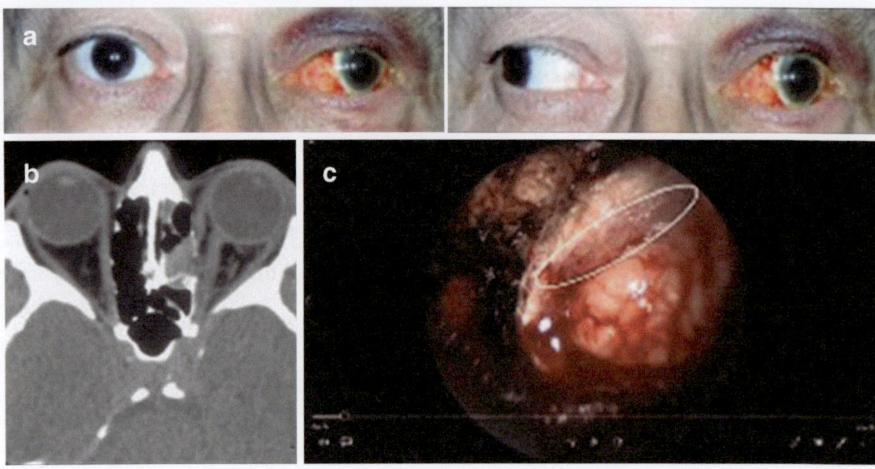

Fig. 3.1 Postoperative and intraoperative findings. (**a**) These photos depict the postoperative physical exam findings. Note in the photo on the left the patient's periorbital ecchymosis, chemosis, and subconjunctival hemorrhage. During straight-ahead gaze there is lateral deviation of the left globe due to injury to the left medial rectus muscle. The photo on the right displays the patient's inability to adduct his left eye due to a medial rectus muscle injury. (**b**) This axial CT displays the patient's injury to the left medial orbital wall. Note how the medial rectus muscle is transected at the site of the injury. There is also a medial displacement of the optic nerve dangerously close to the site of injury. (**c**) This is an intraoperative photo taken during left-sided sinus surgery. In this image, the medial orbital wall has been removed revealing the medial rectus running obliquely (*white circle*) and intraorbital fat below. Indiscriminate use of powered instrumentation along the medial orbital wall can cause rapid tissue removal, leading to significant orbital injuries. Careful identification of abnormal looking structures should be immediately noted and surgical dissection should be stopped

Root Cause Analysis

In the patient described above, the complication could have been avoided at multiple stages during the surgery. Preoperative review of the anatomy would have identified the medial portion of the superior oblique in the anterior ethmoid artery foramen as well as the close proximity of the medial rectus to an already thinned medial orbital wall due to compression necrosis from long-standing nasal polyposis. Intraoperatively, early identification of the lamina would have allowed for preservation of its integrity. Bleeding, which is common during polypectomy, could have been managed with preoperative oral steroids in the immediate days prior to surgery, the use of total intravenous sedation, elevation of the head of the bed, warm saline irrigations, and topical application of vasoconstrictive agents such as epinephrine or oxymetazoline. When normal anatomical landmarks became obscured, the use of image guidance to confirm location and or changing locations from an unfamiliar to known location could have prevented inadvertent debridement of the extraocular muscles.

Lessons Learned

Endoscopic sinus surgery is the standard surgical treatment for medically resistant chronic rhinosinusitis. While statistically rare, complications of endoscopic sinus surgery have the potential to be devastating and even life threatening. Major complications include orbital complications, intracranial complications, and massive hemorrhage. The overall major complication rate in the United States is estimated to be 1%, with orbital injury making up 0.07% of these injuries [1]. When injuries occur to the extraocular muscles, the most commonly involved muscle is the medial rectus and the most common entry point into the orbit is the lower medial orbital wall in the middle to posterior portion of the ethmoid cavity [2–4]. The resulting strabismus from extraocular muscle injury can rarely be resolved even with surgery, and the absence of diplopia with central gaze is frequently the best result a patient can get. In the case illustrated above, the patient suffered an injury to the left medial rectus and superior oblique muscles during polypectomy with powered instrumentation. This occurred during the left-sided maxillary antrostomy and ethmoidectomy portion of the procedure.

In order to better understand how to avoid injuries such as the one this patient experienced, it is imperative to appreciate several key points. First, the anatomy of the orbit is cone shaped, such that it is wider anteriorly and narrows posteriorly. As such, the proximity of the extraocular muscles changes in relationship to the medial orbital wall in an anterior to posterior direction. Anteriorly, the medial and inferior recti as well as the superior oblique are further away from the medial orbital wall and protected by fat whereas posteriorly they are more intimately associated with the medial orbital wall, without intervening fat (Figs. 3.2 and 3.3). Additionally, at

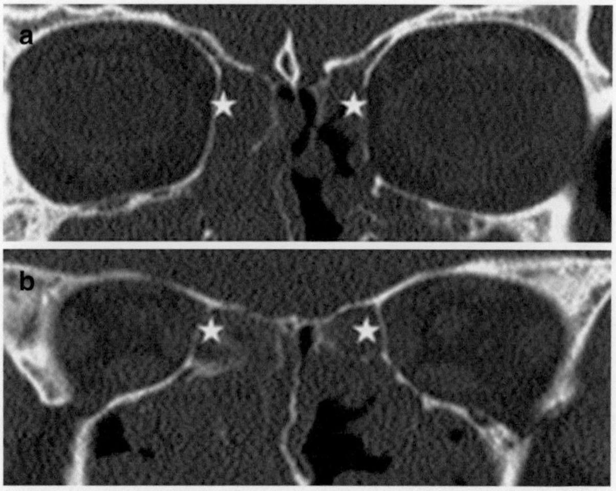

Fig. 3.2 Coronal CT showing relative relationships between the extraocular muscles and the medial orbital wall. (**a**) This image depicts the relationship found in the anterior orbit. Note there is a cushion of fat between the medial orbital wall and the extraocular muscles (*white stars*). (**b**) This image depicts the relationship found in the posterior orbit at the level of the posterior ethmoid cavity. Note close approximation of the extraocular muscles to the medial orbital wall with little intervening fat (*white stars*)

the location of the anterior ethmoid artery's entrance into the nasal cavity, there can be an omega-shaped wedge of bone protruding into the sinonasal cavity, classically called the "nipple sign." In some patients, this foramen can contain a portion of the superior oblique muscle (Fig. 3.4). If bleeding from artery injury were to occur in this area, application of cautery, even bipolar cautery, could potentially cause muscle injury.

Second, the use of powered instrumentation during FESS, while overall safe, when misplaced into the orbit can lead to major ophthalmic complications including extraocular muscle injury, optic nerve damage or even enucleation [5–8]. While the microdebrider has revolutionized endoscopic sinus surgery, the indiscriminate aspirating function, accelerated tissue resection compared to conventional instrumentation and limited tactile feedback can lead to rapid surgical complications [6, 8]. In a cadaveric study by Worden et al., microdebriders were utilized to simulate ophthalmic injuries during FESS, and they found that the average time from violation of periorbita to complete transection of the medial rectus took only 13.4 s, with a minimum time of 4 s [8].

Preoperative strategies to minimize extraocular muscle injury should include a thorough history and physical. Key history points such as primary orbital pathology, facial trauma, sinonasal neoplasm, or endonasal procedures should heighten the surgeon's suspicion for potential compromise of the lamina. A lack of understanding of patient-specific anatomy can lead to complications that may otherwise have been avoidable. Poor preoperative imaging quality and lack of familiarity with

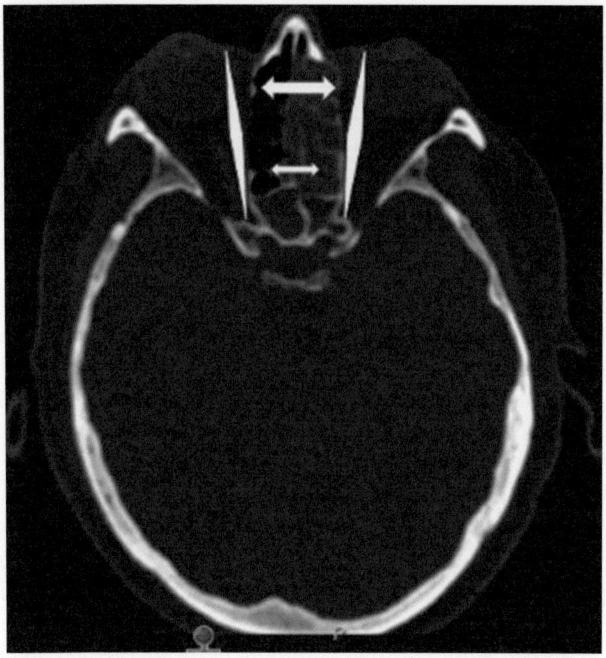

Fig. 3.3 Relative relationship between the medial rectus muscle and the medial orbital wall. Axial CT showing relative relationships between the medial rectus muscles (*white diamonds*) and the medial orbital walls. The *large, double-sided white arrow* is positioned in the anterior ethmoid cavities, and the *small double-sided white arrow* is positioned in the posterior ethmoid cavities. Note the differences in distance between the medial recti and the medial orbital walls anteriorly and posteriorly. An injury to the medial orbital wall posteriorly has a higher likelihood of causing extraocular muscle complications due to direct muscle injury or resultant bleeding putting pressure on the extraocular muscles or optic nerve

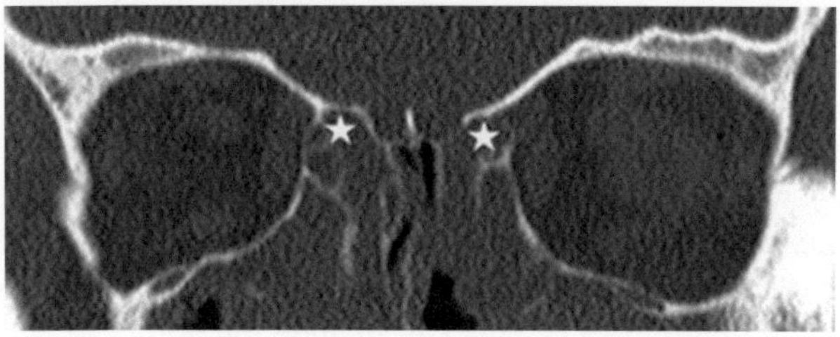

Fig. 3.4 Anteriorethmoid artery foramen and its association with the superior oblique. Coronal CT image displaying classic "nipple sign" of the anterior ethmoid artery foramen entering into the sinonasal cavity. Note how the superior oblique muscles protrude into the foramina (*white stars*). Violation of the anterior ethmoid artery foramen at this location could cause significant bleeding or direct injury to the superior oblique muscle or its trochlea. Careless attempts to cauterize bleeding in this area could also cause muscle injury

computed tomography (CT) can similarly contribute. Thin cut sections, a minimum of 3 mm or thinner (ideally 1 mm or less), reformatted in coronal and sagittal planes set to bone windowing allow for fine detail assessment. The use of a preoperative surgical checklist allows for detailed analysis of the preoperative imaging and can cue the surgeon in to potential pitfalls such as preexisting dehiscence of the orbit with prolapse of orbital contents into the ethmoid cavity. Additional considerations with regard to the sinuses and their relationship to the orbit include the assessing of the overall shape of the lamina, asymmetries of the orientation of the lamina, the location of the anterior ethmoid artery and its relationship to the skull base and superior oblique muscle, the position and rotation of the uncinate process with respect to the orbital wall, as well as the presence of infraorbital ethmoid (Haller) cells. A detailed assessment of the patient's preoperative anatomy allows the surgeon to have a mental roadmap to refer to throughout surgery as well as facilitate identification of potential danger zones as surgery progresses.

Intraoperatively, it is paramount to identify and completely skeletonize the medial orbital wall early, as this will serve as a marker for the lateral most limit of the dissection and allow for protection of the orbital contents. If the medial orbital wall has been adequately skeletonized, a blunt instrument can be used to apply gentle lateral pressure along the medial orbital wall and the entire wall will move as a unit. If residual ethmoid partitions remain, there will be only focal movement or no movement at all [9]. After the lower ethmoid cells are opened and the sphenoidotomy is completed with identification of the skull base, the dissection of the superior cells is then performed posterior to anterior. Using the medial orbital wall and skull base as a guide, the dissection can be completed in a safe and efficient manner. Meticulous and judicious dissection is the key. As the surgery proceeds along the lamina, the force should be directed anteriorly and parallel to the face of the lamina [3]. This prevents inadvertent penetration of the orbit. Great care should be taken when using the microdebrider along the lamina. The cutting side of the blade should be under direct visualization and never be forcefully pressed onto the lamina. If the microdebrider is being used in an area of concern or unclear anatomy, it should be activated in short bursts to avoid the rapid removal of large tissue volumes [3]. If the lamina is violated and orbital contents exposed, immediately terminate dissection in that area. Do not manipulate or remove fat, as this can cause muscle injury or tear bridging vessels with resultant retrobulbar hematoma. Gentle bipolaring of the herniated orbital fat can be used to tease the fat back and allow continued access to the sinuses to finish the procedure. If an inadvertent injury does occur, have a rapid and effective treatment plan in place. This can include the ability to perform a lateral canthotomy and cantholysis if a rapid increase in intraorbital pressure is suspected. The patient should be intraoperatively and postoperatively monitored for signs of serious orbital hematoma, including lid edema, periorbital ecchymosis, proptosis, and firmness of the orbital contents on palpation. Ethmoid packing should be limited to avoid placing pressure on the exposed intraorbital contents. Postoperatively, the patient should be assessed for vision changes including diplopia or vision loss, with referrals to ophthalmology as appropriate.

Extraocular muscle injury, while uncommon, can lead to devastating postoperative complications.

Preoperative preparation, including a checklist and careful review of patient anatomy, is key to a successful surgery. Understanding the danger zones when operating near the orbit as well as the dissection techniques required to safely perform tissue removal in this area are critical to improve outcomes.

References

1. Ramakrishnan VR, Kingdom TT, Nayak JV, Hwang PH, Orlandi RR. Nationwide incidence of major complications in endoscopic sinus surgery. Int Forum Allergy Rhinol. 2012;2(1):34–9.
2. Thacker NM, Velez FG, Demer JL, Wang MB, Rosenbaum AL. Extraocular muscle damage associated with endoscopic sinus surgery: an ophthalmology perspective. Am J Rhinol Provid. 2005;19(4):400–5.
3. Bleier BS, Schlosser RJ. Prevention and management of medial rectus injury. Otolaryngol Clin N Am. 2010;43(4):801–7.
4. Bhatti MT, Schmalfuss IM, Mancuso AA. Orbital complications of functional endoscopic sinus surgery: MR and CT findings. Clin Radiol. 2005;60(8):894–904.
5. Ferguson BJ, DiBiase PA, D'Amico F. Quantitative analysis of microdebriders used in endoscopic sinus surgery. Am J Otolaryngol. 1999;20(5):294–7.
6. Tang D, Lobo BC, D'Anza B, Woodard TD, Sindwani R. Advances in Microdebrider technology: improving functionality and expanding utility. Otolaryngol Clin N Am. 2017;50(3):589–98.
7. Chang JR, Grant MP, Merbs SL. Enucleation as endoscopic sinus surgery complication. JAMA Ophthalmol. 2015;133(7):850–2.
8. Worden CP, Clark CA, Senior AK, Schlosser RJ, Kimple AJ, Senior BA. Modeling Microdebrider-mediated ophthalmic damage: a word of caution in endoscopic sinus surgery. Rhinol Online. 2019;2:44–9.
9. Shah RR, Thomas WW, Kuan EC, Kennedy DW. The lamina push test: an alternative to the globe push test for identifying the medial orbit during endoscopic sinus surgery. Int Forum Allergy Rhinol. 2018;8(9):1073–5.

Chapter 4
Lacrimal Injury During Endoscopic Sinus Surgery: Avoidance and Management

Daniel M. Beswick and Todd T. Kingdom

Pearls

1. Aggressive takedown of the uncinate process is one common cause of nasolacrimal duct (NLD) injury during endoscopic sinus surgery due to the intimate relationship of the nasolacrimal system and lateral nasal wall.
2. The majority of patients remain asymptomatic following NLD injury. Therefore, if NLD injury occurs, further dissection near the site of injury should generally be minimized to limit scarring and preserve the option for future formal dacryocystorhinostomy (DCR).
3. For patients who develop persistent postoperative epiphora, close monitoring, consultation with an ophthalmologist, and additional testing to evaluate the nasolacrimal system are important.
4. Patients with persistent epiphora and NLD obstruction after NLD injury are candidates for DCR.

D. M. Beswick
Department of Head and Neck Surgery, University of California, Los Angeles, Los Angeles, CA, USA

T. T. Kingdom (✉)
Department of Otolaryngology – Head and Neck Surgery, University of Colorado, Aurora, CO, USA

Department of Ophthalmology, University of Colorado, Aurora, CO, USA
e-mail: Todd.Kingdom@cuanschutz.edu

R. K. Chandra, K. C. Welch (eds.), *Lessons Learned from Rhinologic Procedure Complications*, https://doi.org/10.1007/978-3-030-75323-8_4

Case Presentation

A 41-year-old female was referred to our rhinology service after prior endoscopic sinus surgery (ESS). Her medical history was significant for chronic rhinosinusitis (CRS) and allergic rhinitis. Postoperatively, she developed left-sided epiphora that did not resolve for 2 months and had persistent symptoms related to CRS. Endoscopic examination revealed an injury to the left nasolacrimal duct (NLD) at the level of the head of the middle turbinate. This was confirmed on computed tomography (CT) scan (Fig. 4.1), which also demonstrated ongoing sinus inflammation. Evaluation by the ophthalmology service demonstrated NLD obstruction during lacrimal irrigation. After a discussion of treatment options, the patient proceeded with endoscopic DCR (Fig. 4.2) and revision sinus surgery, which resolved the epiphora and other symptoms.

Root Cause Analysis

The nasolacrimal system facilitates drainage of tears and is composed of the lacrimal gland; superior, inferior, and common canaliculi; nasolacrimal sac (NLS); and NLD [1]. The surgeon must appreciate the close anatomical relationships between the NLS and NLD with structures commonly dissected along the lateral nasal wall during ESS, as well as other procedures including endoscopic or open medial maxillectomy, inferior turbinate surgery, and maxillary fracture repair [2–5]. During ESS, uncinectomy and maxillary antrostomy are among the most likely procedures to cause NLD injury. This stems from the positional relationship of the NLS and NLD to the maxillary line, which has been described intranasally as the junction of

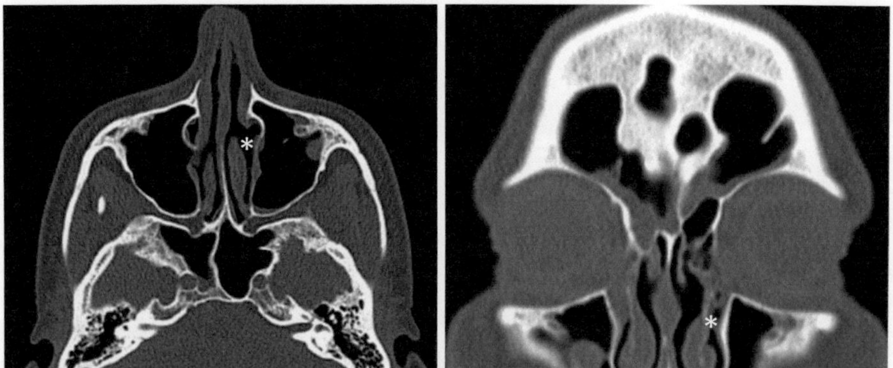

Fig. 4.1 Axial (left) and coronal (right) computed tomography images demonstrating previous injury to the left nasolacrimal duct. The asterisk identifies the site of injury

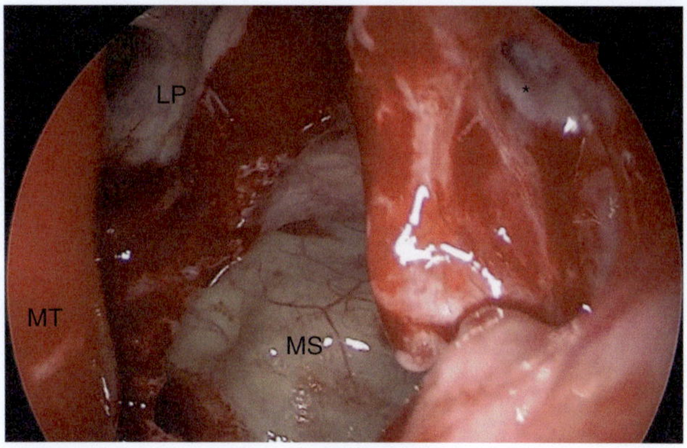

Fig. 4.2 Left nasal endoscopy image during revision endoscopic sinus surgery demonstrating prior injury to nasolacrimal duct, presumably during takedown of the uncinate process. MS: maxillary sinus, MT: middle turbinate, *: opening into left nasolacrimal duct, LP: lamina papyracea

the uncinate process and frontal process of the maxilla, and is at times used as a landmark during ESS [2, 6]. While many cases of NLD injury may remain asymptomatic postoperatively, disruption of the NLD can cause subsequent obstruction, epiphora, dacryocystitis, and/or scarring.

In addition to appreciating a specific patient's anatomy through CT scan analysis, a broad and detailed understanding of lateral nasal wall anatomy in general is important. The NLS extends, on average, 8.8 ± 0.2 mm above and 4.1 ± 2.3 mm below the insertion of the middle turbinate on the lateral nasal wall [7]. The NLD extends inferiorly from the NLS and has an intraosseous portion and intrameatal portion, the latter of which is located lateral to the inferior turbinate and drains through Hasner's valve [8]. Cadaveric studies have shown the distance from the alar rim to the NLD to be 4.1–4.3 ± 0.5 cm and determined the nearest distance from the natural os of the maxillary sinus to the posterior aspect of the NLD to be 4.0 ± 1.2 mm [2, 9]. Variation in distances and anatomy exists, and it is important to use these measurements as estimates. Additionally, the maxillary line and NLD have a variable positional relationship; studies have demonstrated that the maxillary line can be posterior to, anterior to, or overlapping with the NLD [2, 9]. A more consistent relationship between the NLD and lateral wall structures is found using the free, posterior edge of the uncinate process, which is posterior to the NLD [1, 2, 10].

Lessons Learned

Avoidance

Knowledge and recognition of nasal landmarks are the foundation of avoiding NLD injury during endoscopic sinus surgery. Estimates of the distance from landmarks to the NLD are helpful in surgical planning; however, these alone are insufficient and each case must be evaluated individually focusing on preoperative CT imaging. The size, shape, orientation, and bony covering or absence thereof of the NLD should be evaluated, along with the other standard features of a preoperative CT before ESS. During ESS, the NLD is most at risk during uncinectomy and maxillary antrostomy. Additional procedures and approaches, such as surgery for neoplasms, endoscopic modified medial maxillectomy, and prelacrimal techniques, may increase the likelihood of NLD injury, though the overall risk of injury to this structure remains low when good surgical technique is practiced. Commonly adhered to techniques to avoid NLD injury include avoiding aggressive takedown of the uncinate process and, when endoscopic modified medial maxillectomy is performed, ensuring that the anterior component of medial maxillary wall removal is performed inferior to Hasner's valve.

Assessment and Management of NLD Injury

NLD injury is often asymptomatic, but surgeons must be prepared to manage possible symptomatic consequences as unintended violation of the NLD during ESS can lead to scarring and epiphora. Studies have suggested that epiphora is reported following 0.1–1.7% of cases of ESS [11–15]; however, these original studies are from 2–4 decades ago when complications occurred more frequently compared to today, and the rates of NLD injury and epiphora are likely lower in the current era. Epiphora, when it occurs following NLD injury, most commonly presents within 2–3 weeks of surgery and may resolve over subsequent weeks as intranasal inflammation subsides [1, 16].

When NLD injury occurs during ESS and is recognized intraoperatively, several strategies can be employed. Generally, minimizing further dissection around the site of injury will limit postoperative scarring. As NLD injury commonly happens near the midportion of the duct during takedown of the uncinate process, limiting additional superior dissection also preserves the option for traditional dacryocystorhinostomy (DCR) at a later date, if needed. A wait-and-watch approach is supported by the fact that many instances of NLD injury are either asymptomatic or associated with spontaneous resolution of epiphora, should epiphora develop postoperatively. Another option involves intraoperative consultation to the ophthalmology service with consideration of lacrimal intubation or stenting. The rate of spontaneous recovery after NLD injury is unknown; thus, evidence-based guidelines for intraoperative management are lacking.

Patients who sustained NLD injury and those who develop epiphora postoperatively warrant close monitoring. If epiphora resolves within several weeks, these patients can often be observed without additional testing. Persistent epiphora necessitates additional workup to evaluate the nasolacrimal system, which is often performed in conjunction with an ophthalmologist. Schirmer's test, while more commonly employed for dry eye, can be utilized to assess for NLD obstruction. This test involves placing a filter paper strip near the middle portion of the lower eyelid and measuring the length of tear collection on the strip after 5 minutes; values >30 mm are suggestive of NLD obstruction. Fluorescein dye instilled in the inferior fornix should be absent after 10 minutes due to the natural turnover time of lacrimal film. Abnormalities in these two tests can establish if NLD obstruction is present though do not specify the site of obstruction. Additional clinical tests that provide more detail about the site of obstruction include lacrimal irrigation, Jones I test, and Jones II test. Radiographic studies, including fluoroscopic dacryocystogram, lacrimal scintigraphy, and CT are available options to supplement clinical tests but are not commonly required [17].

For persistent, symptomatic epiphora following NLD injury, DCR is an option for patients and typically has high success rates, >85% [1, 16, 17]. DCR can be performed via external or endonasal approaches, with results thought to be similar between approaches [18]. DCR is best suited to treat obstruction of the NLD or the inferior nasolacrimal sac; this procedure alone will not improve more proximal obstructions, such as those that involve the canaliculus.

Conclusion

Thorough anatomical knowledge of the nasolacrimal system and lateral nasal wall minimizes the risk of injury to the NLD during ESS. Careful evaluation of preoperative imaging can further decrease this risk, as anatomical variations are common and must be identified preoperatively. NLD injury during ESS is rare and most patients who sustain this injury will remain asymptomatic postoperatively. For those patients who develop persistent epiphora following surgery, ongoing monitoring, consultation with an ophthalmologist, and further testing to evaluate the nasolacrimal system are indicated. DCR is a treatment option for persistent epiphora after NLD injury and has good outcomes.

Disclosures/Potential Conflicts of Interest DMB: Medtronic, consultant not affiliated with this work (ended 2020); TTK: none.

References

1. Cohen NA, Antunes MB, Morgenstern KE. Prevention and management of lacrimal duct injury. Otolaryngol Clin N Am. 2010;43:781–8.
2. Ali MJ, Nayak JV, Vaezeafshar R, Li G, Psaltis AJ. Anatomic relationship of nasolacrimal duct and major lateral wall landmarks: cadaveric study with surgical implications. Int Forum Allergy Rhinol. 2014;4:684–8.
3. Imre A, Imre SS, Pinar E, et al. Transection of nasolacrimal duct in endoscopic medial Maxillectomy: implication on Epiphora. J Craniofac Surg. 2015;26:e616–9.
4. Shoshani Y, Samet N, Ardekian L, Taicher S. Nasolacrimal duct injury after Le Fort I osteotomy. J Oral Maxillofac Surg. 1994;52:406–7.
5. Unlu HH, Goktan C, Aslan A, Tarhan S. Injury to the lacrimal apparatus after endoscopic sinus surgery: surgical implications from active transport dacryocystography. Otolaryngol Head Neck Surg. 2001;124:308–12.

6. Chastain JB, Cooper MH, Sindwani R. The maxillary line: anatomic characterization and clinical utility of an important surgical landmark. Laryngoscope. 2005;115:990–2.
7. Wormald PJ, Kew J, Van Hasselt A. Intranasal anatomy of the nasolacrimal sac in endoscopic dacryocystorhinostomy. Otolaryngol Head Neck Surg. 2000;123:307–10.
8. Burkat CN, Lucarelli MJ. Anatomy of the lacrimal system. New York: Springer. 2006
9. Kim YH, Park MG, Kim GC, Park BS, Kwak HH. Topography of the nasolacrimal duct on the lateral nasal wall in Koreans. Surg Radiol Anat. 2012;34:249–55.
10. Calhoun KH, Rotzler WH, Stiernberg CM. Surgical anatomy of the lateral nasal wall. Otolaryngol Head Neck Surg. 1990;102:156–60.
11. Bolger WE, Parsons DS, Mair EA, Kuhn FA. Lacrimal drainage system injury in functional endoscopic sinus surgery. Incidence, analysis, and prevention. Arch Otolaryngol Head Neck Surg. 1992;118:1179–84.
12. Davis WE, Templer JW, Lamear WR, Davis WE Jr, Craig SB. Middle meatus anstrostomy: patency rates and risk factors. Otolaryngol Head Neck Surg. 1991;104:467–72.
13. Freedman HM, Kern EB. Complications of intranasal ethmoidectomy: a review of 1,000 consecutive operations. Laryngoscope. 1979;89:421–34.
14. Kennedy DW, Zinreich SJ, Shaalan H, Kuhn F, Naclerio R, Loch E. Endoscopic middle meatal antrostomy: theory, technique, and patency. Laryngoscope. 1987;97:1–9.
15. Unlu HH, Govsa F, Mutlu C, Yuceturk AV, Senyilmaz Y. Anatomical guidelines for intranasal surgery of the lacrimal drainage system. Rhinology. 1997;35:11–5.
16. Hosemann W, Draf C. Danger points, complications and medico-legal aspects in endoscopic sinus surgery. GMS Curr Top Otorhinolaryngol Head Neck Surg. 2013;12:Doc06.
17. Kingdom TT, Barham HP, Durairaj VD. Long-term outcomes after endoscopic dacryocystorhinostomy without mucosal flap preservation. Laryngoscope. 2020;130:12–7.
18. Jawaheer L, MacEwen CJ, Anijeet D. Endonasal versus external dacryocystorhinostomy for nasolacrimal duct obstruction. Cochrane Database Syst Rev. 2017;2:CD007097.

Chapter 5
Orbital Complications: Nasolacrimal Duct Injury After Endoscopic Sinus Surgery

Dennis M. Tang and Raj Sindwani

Clinical Pearls

1. Carefully identify the maxillary line as the key landmark for the location of the nasolacrimal duct along the lateral nasal wall.
2. Exercise caution when enlarging a maxillary antrostomy anteriorly, especially when using heavy instruments like the backbiting forceps.
3. Consider dacryocystorhinostomy for the management of verified nasolacrimal duct injuries following sinus surgery.

Case Presentation

Patient is a 54-year-old male, previously healthy, who was referred for chronic rhinosinusitis. He was previously treated by his primary care physician with intranasal steroids and antibiotics. He continued to complain of nasal congestion and cheek tenderness. A computed tomography (CT) scan was obtained that showed a unilateral left maxillary sinus mass with no bony erosion. On presentation, the patient was noted to have a unilateral mass protruding from the middle meatus. An in-clinic biopsy was consistent with sinonasal papilloma – inverted type (IP).

D. M. Tang
Department of Otolaryngology, Cedars-Sinai Medical Center, Los Angeles, CA, USA

R. Sindwani (✉)
Section of Rhinology, Sinus, and Skull Base Surgery, Head and Neck Institute, Cleveland Clinic, Cleveland, OH, USA

Minimally Invasive Cranial Base and Pituitary Surgery, Rosa Ella Burkhardt Brain Tumor & Neuro-Oncology Center, Cleveland Clinic, Cleveland, OH, USA
e-mail: Sindwar@ccf.org

R. K. Chandra, K. C. Welch (eds.), *Lessons Learned from Rhinologic Procedure Complications*, https://doi.org/10.1007/978-3-030-75323-8_5

He was taken to the operating room and underwent an endoscopic medial maxillectomy and removal of the IP. It appeared to be pedunculated just posterior to the zygomatic recess. A medial maxillectomy was performed taking the middle portion of the inferior turbinate. The medial wall was removed anteriorly to the maxillary line using a drill and back-biting forceps. Angled scopes and instruments were used to remove the mass in its entirety. An angled diamond burr was then used to drill the underlying bone at the site of attachment.

At the 3-week postoperative follow-up, the patient noticed worsening epiphora in his left eye. He constantly carried tissues around for his tearing and was quite bothered by it. On examination, his left eye appeared more tear-laden compared to the right. Nasal endoscopy revealed a well-healed postoperative maxillary sinus cavity. A referral to ophthalmology was pursued. A slit lamp examination revealed an elevated tear lake on the left. The ophthalmologist performed probing and irrigation and noted to have increased resistance with reflux from both punctae, suggestive of a distal nasolacrimal duct obstruction.

After 3 months of persistent symptoms, the patient agreed to surgery and he was taken back to the operating room and an endoscopic dacryocystorhinostomy (E-DCR) was performed. A Crawford stent was placed. The patient had immediate and sustained resolution of his left-sided epiphora. The stent was removed in the clinic after 4 weeks with no recurrence of epiphora.

Root Cause Analysis

This patient suffered the complication of a nasolacrimal duct (NLD) injury after sinus surgery, likely due to failure to identify this structure and its anatomic course intraoperatively. The exact incidence of this is unknown. Historically, occult injury is thought to occur between 3% and 15% of all endoscopic sinus surgeries (ESS); however, modern rates may be much lower than this [1, 2]. Frequently, intraoperative injury to the NLD can heal spontaneously and clinical sequelae are rare [2]. The NLD is located in the anterior portion of the medial maxillary wall (Fig. 5.1). One would expect that the incidence would be higher for procedures that create a larger antrostomy and expanded approaches such as the endoscopic medial maxillectomy highlighted in the case presented.

The key landmark for the location of the NLD endoscopically is the maxillary line that corresponds to the junction of the uncinate and maxilla [3]. Extranasally, the maxillary line correlates with the suture line between the lacrimal bone and the frontal process of the maxilla [4]. Injury to the nasolacrimal canal (and the duct it contains) can occur during anterior enlargement of the maxillary antrostomy (Fig. 5.2). An anatomic study showed that lacrimal duct penetration occurs at a mean distance of 3.7 mm posterior to the maxillary line with no penetration occurring at a minimum distance of 7 mm posterior to the maxillary line [5]. Therefore, care should be exercised as one removes the last portion of the uncinate process where it articulates at the maxillary line and when the maxillary ostium is enlarged

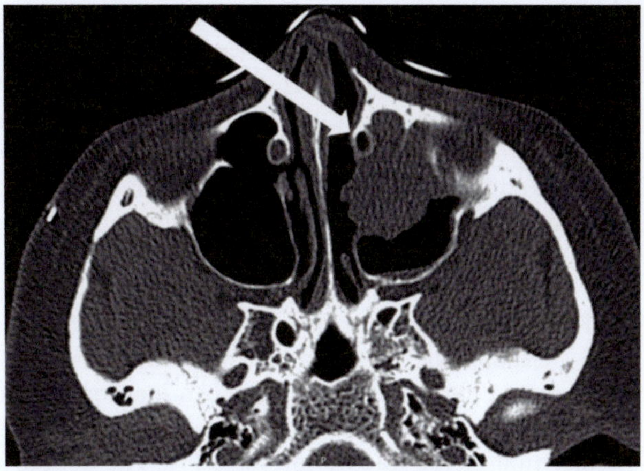

Fig. 5.1 CT axial scan with arrow indicating position of left nasolacrimal duct in close proximity to the left maxillary sinus inverted papilloma

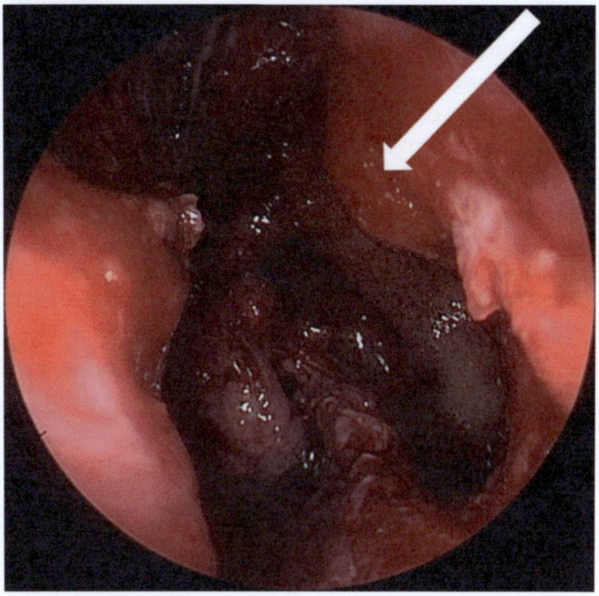

Fig. 5.2 Endoscopic view of left nasal cavity with arrow indication position of left nasolacrimal duct at the edge of the anterior medial maxillectomy margin

in the anterior dimension, especially when heavier instruments such as backbiting forceps are used.

Patients who present with epiphora after ESS should have a complete ophthalmologic evaluation. Previously, the method of identifying the level of obstruction was performed via Jones tests. In the Jones I test, fluorescein is placed in the conjunctival sac and recovered using a cotton-tip applicator in the inferior meatus. Recovery of fluorescein in the inferior meatus is considered a positive test while failure to recover dye is considered a negative test. If the Jones I test is negative, a Jones II test is performed where the inferior canaliculus is cannulated and irrigated with clear saline. Presence of fluorescein in the solution indicates that a patent canalicular system is intact with a partially obstructed lower system. Recovery of clear fluid without fluorescein indicates a dysfunctional canalicular system. Another method of identifying the level of obstruction is through lacrimal irrigation test. In the lacrimal irrigation test, the lacrimal puncta is cannulated and irrigation is performed. Recovery of irrigation in the nose indicates a patent or partially patent system. Reflux through the same canaliculus indicates obstruction of that canaliculus. Reflux through the opposite canaliculus indicates common canaliculus obstruction. Distension of the nasolacrimal sac indicates nasolacrimal duct obstruction.

Management of NLD injury after ESS can be through a dacryocystorhinostomy (DCR). This can be performed via an open approach or an endoscopic approach. In the E-DCR approach, the lacrimal sac is landmarked using the axilla of the middle turbinate and the maxillary line [6]. An incision is made anterior to the sac and a mucosal flap is elevated. The sac has been shown on average to extend 8 mm above the insertion of the middle turbinate [7]. The bone overlying the sac is removed using a high-speed drill or Kerrison punch forceps creating a bony window of 10–12 mm in diameter. Once the bone is removed, an incision is made using a sickle or arachnoid knife into the sac as its medial wall is tented using a lacrimal probe placed externally through the canalicular system (Fig. 5.3). This opening is enlarged using through-cut forceps or a microdebrider such that the entire medial sac wall is resected. The previously raised mucosal flap can be used to line the tract if preferred, although the necessity of this flap technique is debated. Stents or tubes are placed through the superior and inferior canaliculus if desired. The timing of removal of these stents varies, but typically range between 3 and 8 weeks and can be performed in the office.

The endoscopic DCR technique is a very well-tolerated outpatient procedure. Compared to the traditional open approach to DCR, the E-DCR avoids an external incision on the face and the resultant scar. Postoperative care is similar to ESS, with patients instructed to begin saline irrigations on postoperative day #1. Complications of E-DCR can include ecchymosis, orbital fat exposure, re-stenosis (failure),

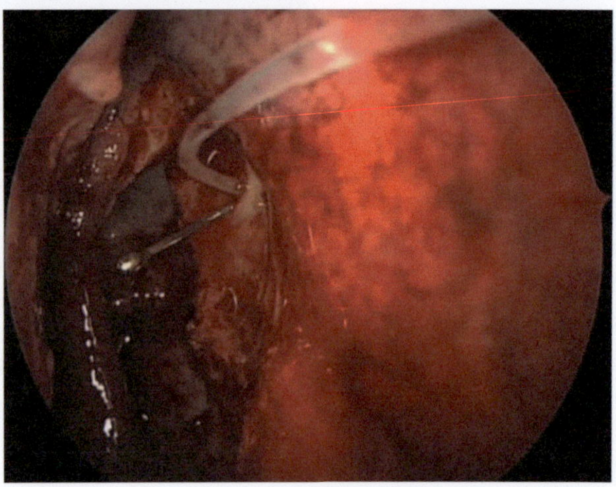

Fig. 5.3 Endoscopic view of the left nasal cavity with lacrimal stent in place during an endoscopic dacryocystorhinostomy

intraorbital injury, and lacerations to the inferior canaliculus. Success rates in the literature range from 87% to 98%, with recent meta-analyses establishing that mechanical (nonlaser) endoscopic DCRs have equivalent success rates to traditional open techniques [8].

Lessons Learned

Intraoperative iatrogenic injury to the NLD during endoscopic ESS is a known entity, although clinical sequelae are rare. Injuries to the NLD can occur during anterior enlargement of the maxillary antrostomy. Anatomical knowledge of the location and course of the lacrimal apparatus is critical. When suspected, the patient should undergo a complete ophthalmologic evaluation to characterize the location of the injury. A DCR can be performed, which permits tear drainage proximal to the site of injury, and corrects symptoms in the majority of patients [9].

Primary Institution Cleveland Clinic Foundation

References

1. Saengpanich S, Kerekhanjanarong V, Chochaipanichnon L, Supiyaphun P. Nasolacrimal duct injury from microscopic sinus surgery: Preliminary report. J Med Assoc Thail. 2001;84(4):562–5.
2. Bolger WE, Parsons DS, Mair EA, Kuhn FA. Lacrimal Drainage System Injury in Functional Endoscopic Sinus Surgery: Incidence, Analysis, and Prevention. Arch Otolaryngol Neck Surg. 1992;118(11):1179–84. https://doi.org/10.1001/archotol.1992.01880110047011.
3. Chastain JB, Sindwani R. Anatomy of the Orbit, Lacrimal Apparatus, and Lateral Nasal Wall. Otolaryngol Clin North Am. 2006;39(5):855–64. https://doi.org/10.1016/j.otc.2006.07.003.
4. Chastain JB, Cooper MH, Sindwani R. The maxillary line: Anatomic characterization and clinical utility of an important surgical landmark. Laryngoscope. 2005;115(6):990–2. https://doi.org/10.1097/01.MLG.0000163764.01776.10.
5. Sarber KM, O'Connor PD, Doellman MS, et al. Surgical relationship of the nasolacrimal system to the maxillary line: performing safe mega antrostomy. Allergy Rhinol. 2015;6(3):ar.2015.6.0138.https://doi.org/10.2500/ar.2015.6.0138.
6. Woog JJ, Sindwani R. Endoscopic Dacryocystorhinostomy and Conjunctivodacryocystorhinostomy. Otolaryngol Clin North Am. 2006;39(5):1001–17. https://doi.org/10.1016/j.otc.2006.08.005.
7. Wormald PJ, Kew J, Van Hasselt A. Intranasal anatomy of the nasolacrimal sac in endoscopic dacryocystorhinostomy. Otolaryngol - Head Neck Surg. 2000;123(3):307–10. https://doi.org/10.1067/mhn.2000.105416.
8. Sobel RK, Aakalu VK, Wladis EJ, Bilyk JR, Yen MT, Mawn LA. A Comparison of Endonasal Dacryocystorhinostomy and External Dacryocystorhinostomy: A Report by the American Academy of Ophthalmology. In: Ophthalmology. Vol 126; 2019:1580–85. https://doi.org/10.1016/j.ophtha.2019.06.009.
9. Cohen NA, Antunes MB, Morgenstern KE. Prevention and management of lacrimal duct injury. Otolaryngol Clin North Am. 2010;43(4):781–8. https://doi.org/10.1016/j.otc.2010.04.005.

Chapter 6
Silent Sinus Syndrome

Ryan E. Little and Rodney J. Schlosser

Clinical Pearls

1. A thoughtful review of the patient's imaging and relevant anatomical considerations are essential to preoperative planning and determination of the appropriate surgical techniques necessary to safely perform surgery in silent sinus syndrome.
2. The instrumentation typically used to perform a retrograde uncinectomy and maxillary antrostomy may not have sufficient lateral reach. Consider utilizing a frontal sinus seeker reverse hook probe to dilate the ethmoid infundibulum and a pediatric backbiter to complete the uncinate resection.
3. It is appropriate to consider the use of intraoperative image guidance technology given the distorted sinus anatomy and ability to register critical landmarks.

Case Presentation

A 45-year-old male with chronic nasal airway obstruction and post-nasal drip was referred to an otolaryngologist for further management. Prior treatment had included topical intranasal steroid sprays and oral antihistamines. There was no prior allergy testing or sinus surgery. He was otherwise asymptomatic from a sinonasal perspective. Preoperative nasal endoscopy noted bilateral inferior turbinate hypertrophy, mild rightward septal deviation and lateralized right middle turbinate with polypoid edema bilaterally. No ophthalmologic nor ophthalmometry examination was obtained preoperatively. Non-contrast sinus CT showed unilateral opacification of the right maxillary sinus with inferior displacement of the orbital floor, inward

R. E. Little (✉) · R. J. Schlosser
Department of Otolaryngology – Head and Neck Surgery, Medical University of South Carolina, Charleston, SC, USA

R. K. Chandra, K. C. Welch (eds.), *Lessons Learned from Rhinologic Procedure Complications*, https://doi.org/10.1007/978-3-030-75323-8_6

bowing of the medial wall of the maxillary sinus and atelectasis of the ethmoid infundibulum (Fig. 6.1).

The patient underwent endoscopic septoplasty, bilateral inferior turbinate reduction, right maxillary antrostomy and right total ethmoidectomy. The operative note reported using a microdebrider to remove inflammatory tissue and polyps within the maxillary and ethmoid cavity. The procedure was halted when atypical bleeding was encountered, and periorbital edema and ecchymosis was noted externally. The operative note reported that intraoperative ophthalmology consultation noted "normal intraocular pressures in the right eye." Postoperatively the patient reported diplopia in primary gaze with an associated outward deviation of the right eye and limited adduction. Postoperative CT and MRI orbits demonstrated violation of the right lamina papyracea, complete transection of the right medial rectus muscle, and disruption of the normal fat planes around the optic nerve (Fig. 6.2). At the patient's 1-week follow-up appointment, he was referred to a local ophthalmologist for persistent ocular motility limitation and consideration of corrective surgery to repair the transected muscle.

Root Cause Analysis

Silent sinus syndrome is a clinical phenomenon characterized by progressive hypoglobus and enophthalmos in association with ipsilateral maxillary sinus collapse in the setting of asymptomatic chronic maxillary sinus hypoventilation [1]. Onset of spontaneous enophthalmos in the setting of chronic maxillary sinusitis was initially described by Montgomery [2]. The term "silent sinus syndrome" was coined by Soparkar et al. and used to describe the asymptomatic and insidious nature of the disease [3, 4].

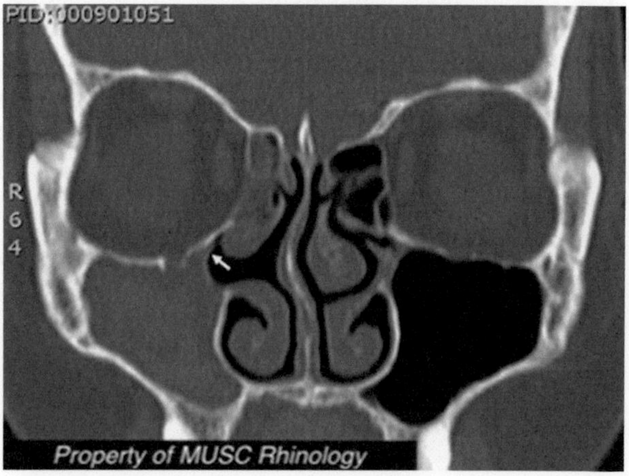

Fig. 6.1 Coronal CT showing silent sinus syndrome involving the right maxillary sinus. Characteristic imaging findings include displacement of the orbital floor, decreased volume of the opacified maxillary sinus and coaptation of the uncinate process juxtaposed to the inferior medial orbital wall (white arrow)

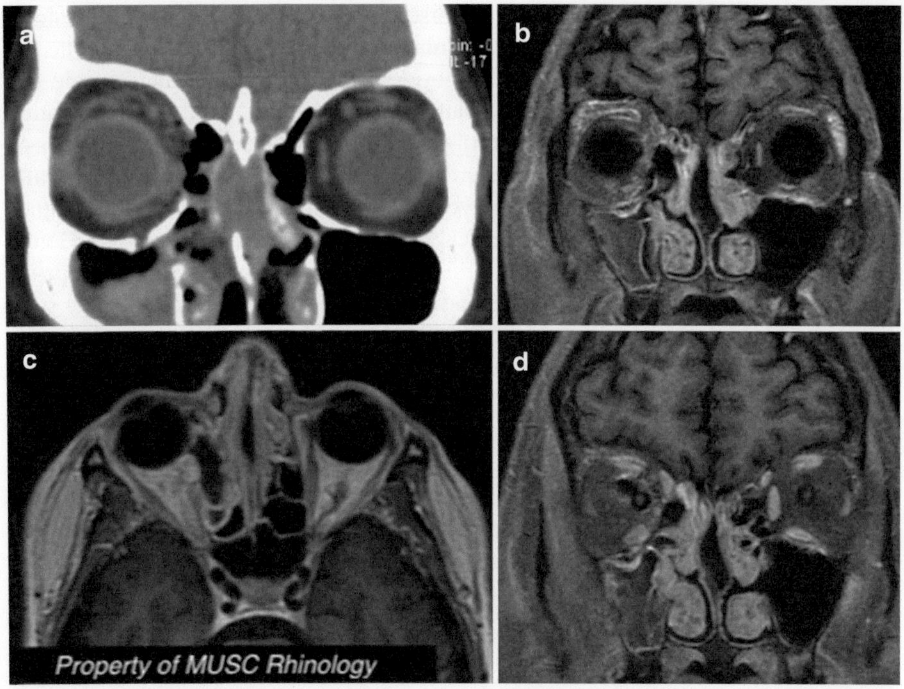

Fig. 6.2 Orbital complication associated with operative treatment of right silent sinus syndrome. CT and MRI imaging modalities showing violation of lamina papyracea, absence of extraconal fat, medial rectus muscle, and intraconal injury in association with the right optic nerve. (**a**) Coronal non-contrast CT; (**b**) coronal MRI T1 contrast enhanced fat suppression; (**c**) axial MRI T1 contrast enhanced; (**d**) coronal MRI T1 contrast enhanced fat suppression

From an endoscopic sinus surgery perspective, a thorough review of preoperative imaging is essential to identifying the unique anatomical considerations and to the prevention of potential operative complications. It is important to recognize changes in maxillary sinus volume and height relative to orbital contents. Additionally, ethmoid infundibulum atelectasis often results in lateralization of the uncinate process, placing the retracted uncinate process in close proximity or direct contact with the lamina papyracea. The astute physician will review CT imaging preoperatively and make the necessary modifications to the surgical technique to avoid ophthalmic complications [5, 6].

Previously reported ophthalmic complications during endoscopic sinus surgery include extraocular muscle, optic nerve, and lamina papyracea damage as well as orbital hematoma and globe penetration [6]. The altered anatomy in silent sinus syndrome places these structures at particular risk of injury [7].

In this case, the first point of note is to recognize chronic maxillary atelectasis (i.e., silent sinus syndrome) in this patient. The second point of note is the failure to detect on the preoperative imaging the narrow ethmoid infundibulum and uncinate relative to the orbit. As a result, the surgical planning and technique necessary for safe uncinectomy in this patient was adversely impacted. Such surgical considerations in silent sinus syndrome include eliminating or significantly limiting the use of the powered microdebrider because debridement of orbital fat and muscle can occur if there is violation of the lamina papyracea. In general, hand instrumentation is favored for the dissection. After optimization of the surgical field with intranasal decongestants, care is taken to identify critical landmarks including the laterally retracted uncinate process. Intraoperative use of computer-aided image guidance technology may be appropriate in cases where the sinus anatomy is distorted. Gentle dilation of atelectatic ethmoid infundibulum using a maxillary ostium seeker probe allows for the uncinectomy to be performed in a retrograde fashion (Fig. 6.3). Anterograde approach using sickle knives or Freer elevators for uncinectomy is generally avoided given the obvious risk of orbital injury. An alternative method for dilating the ethmoid infundibulum utilizes the reverse angle hook on a frontal sinus seeker that can be used to medialize the retracted uncinate and facilitate this dissection. Through-cutting instruments are used to resect the remaining uncinate and posterior fontanelle, taking care when possible to position the working end of the instrument away from the eye. A pediatric backbiter can be helpful in completing the uncinate resection. An angled endoscope may also be used to confirm incorporation of the natural os into the surgical antrostomy. After completion of the maxillary antrostomy, a curved suction is used to evacuate inspissated mucus from the

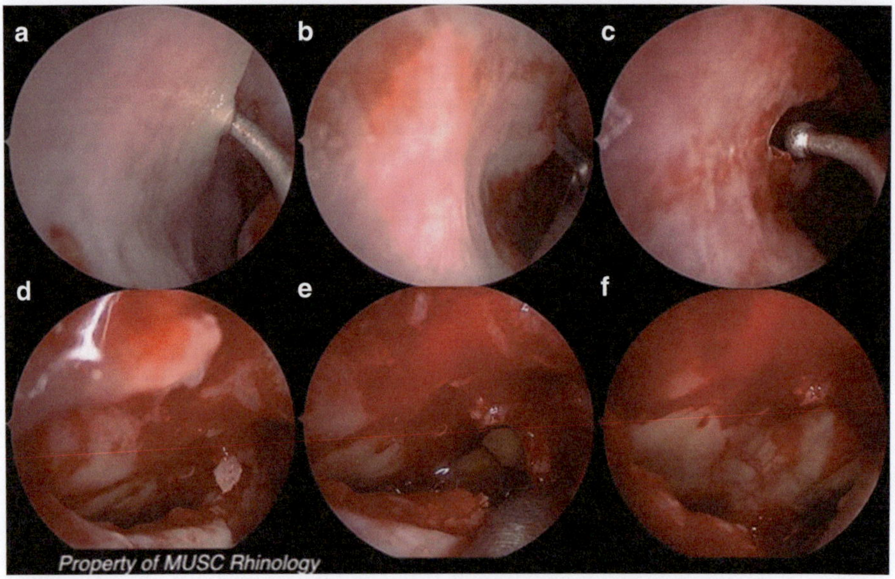

Fig. 6.3 Surgical considerations and technique in silent sinus syndrome. (**a**) Gentle dilation of atelectatic ethmoid infundibulum using a maxillary ostium seeker probe or alternatively a frontal sinus seeker with reverse angle hook; (**b**) uncinotomy performed in retrograde fashion; (**c**) medialization of uncinate to optimize removal; (**d**, **e**) through-cutting instruments are used to retract the uncinate away from the lamina papyracea and resect the remaining uncinate and posterior fontanelle; (**f**) curved suction to evacuate inspissated mucus from the maxillary sinus

maxillary sinus. If retrograde uncinectomy becomes challenging, alternative approaches to enter the maxillary sinus would include entry through the posterior fontanelle or even the inferior meatus. These nonanatomic surgical openings provide orientation to orbital landmarks and then still must be connected to the natural maxillary os.

Lessons Learned

The presentation of silent sinus syndrome can be insidious. There is a greater potential for ophthalmic complications during surgical management of this disease entity than typical endoscopic sinus surgical cases. Keys to avoiding complications are recognition, through careful preoperative imaging review, and intraoperative anatomic correlation, particularly regarding position of the uncinate process.

References

1. Soparkar CN, Patrinely JR, Cuaycong MJ, et al. The silent sinus syndrome. A cause of spontaneous enophthalmos. Ophthalmology. 1994;101:772–8.
2. Montgomery W. Mucocele of the maxillary sinus causing enophthalmos. Eye Ear Nose Throat. 1964;43:41–44.
3. Facon F, Eloy P, Brasseur P, Collet S, Bertrand B. The silent sinus syndrome. Eur Arch Otorhinolaryngol. 2006;263:567–71.
4. Pawar SS, Hong S, Poetker DM. Delayed presentation of silent sinus syndrome after orbital trauma. Am J Otolaryngol. 2010;31:61–3.
5. Numa WA, Desai U, Gold DR, Heher KL, Annino DJ. Silent sinus syndrome: a case presentation and comprehensive review of all 84 reported cases. Ann Otol Rhinol Laryngol. 2005;114:688–94.
6. Vander Meer JB, Harris G, Toohill RJ, Smith TL. The silent sinus syndrome: a case series and literature review. Laryngoscope. 2001;111:975–8.
7. Dunya IM, Salman SD, Shore JW. Ophthalmic complications of endoscopic ethmoid surgery and their management. Am J Otolaryngol. 1996;17:322–31.

Chapter 7
Unusual Orbital Complications of Endoscopic Sinus Surgery

Meha G. Fox and Alexander Chiu

Clinical Pearls

1. Avoid forceful irrigation in the case of extensive disease that may have thinned bony partitions.
2. In a patient with a known bony dehiscence, discuss avoidance of positive pressure mask ventilation with anesthesia colleagues.

Case Presentations

A 56-year-old female presented to the Otolaryngology clinic with symptoms of chronic sinusitis. She was found to have nasal polyposis and purulent secretions draining from the middle meatus. After a course of medical therapy, she elected to proceed with surgical treatment of her disease. Computed tomography (CT) prior to surgery showed a thin lamina papyracea, but no obvious dehiscence on the left side. The patient underwent bilateral maxillary antrostomy, total ethmoidectomy, sphenoidotomy, and frontal sinusotomy. At the end of the procedure, all of the sinuses were irrigated. The frontal sinuses were irrigated with normal saline using a 60 cc syringe connected to a malleable, curved suction. Immediately following irrigation of the left frontal sinus, the patient was noted to have left-sided chemosis (Fig. 7.1).

M. G. Fox (✉)
Department of Otolaryngology-Head and Neck Surgery, Baylor College of Medicine, Houston, TX, USA
e-mail: mgoyal@bcm.edu

A. Chiu
Department of Otolaryngology-Head and Neck Surgery, University of Kansas Medical Center, Kansas City, KS, USA
e-mail: achiu@kumc.edu

R. K. Chandra, K. C. Welch (eds.), *Lessons Learned from Rhinologic Procedure Complications*, https://doi.org/10.1007/978-3-030-75323-8_7

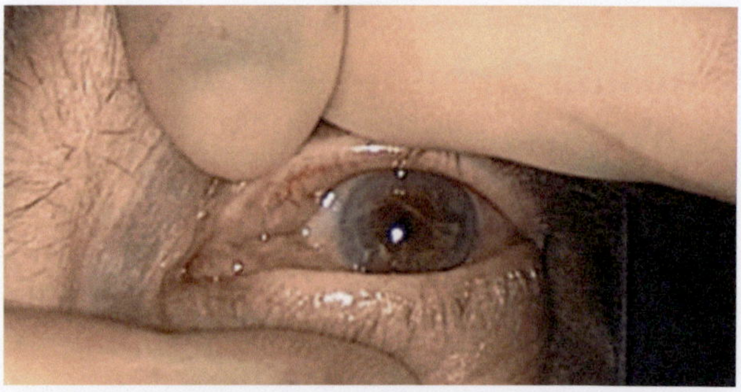

Fig. 7.1 Case 1. Chemosis following endoscopic sinus surgery

Manual massage of the orbit ensued and saline slowly emitted back into the superior ethmoid cavity through a small break in the lamina papyracea. Postoperatively, the patient denied vision changes or orbital pain. She was admitted for overnight observation. Her chemosis completely resolved 3 h postoperatively. She was discharged home the day after surgery and had no long-term sequelae of this complication.

The second case is of a 66-year-old female with chronic rhinosinusitis with nasal polyposis. The patient had undergone prior endoscopic sinus surgery (ESS) and now presented with recurrence of obstructive polyps. Preoperative CT scan showed a small right-sided lamina papyracea dehiscence. She underwent revision bilateral maxillary antrostomy, total ethmoidectomy, sphenoidotomy, and frontal sinusotomy. Intraoperatively, the previous right lamina papyracea defect was identified. Dissection in this area was carried out meticulously in order to avoid further injury to the lamina papyracea and underlying orbital structures. There were no obvious complications during the case. On the first postoperative day, the patient called the clinic due to new-onset diplopia. She was directed to present to the emergency department where a CT scan revealed air in the right orbit (Fig. 7.2). An ophthalmology consult was obtained, and her intra-ocular pressure was within normal limits. She was admitted for observation and her intranasal packing was removed. No additional interventions were pursued. Her diplopia resolved in 48 h. On subsequent postoperative visit, she demonstrated no sequelae of this complication.

Root Cause Analysis

The first orbital complication likely occurred due to a dehiscence of the lamina papyracea and periorbita not appreciable clinically or on imaging. Irrigation under hydrostatic pressure resulted in conjunctival edema. This responded to orbital massage and eventually self-resolved. Furthermore, the patient remained asymptomatic from the complication.

The second patient had a known lamina papyracea dehiscence. She received positive pressure ventilation via bag-valve mask during induction of general

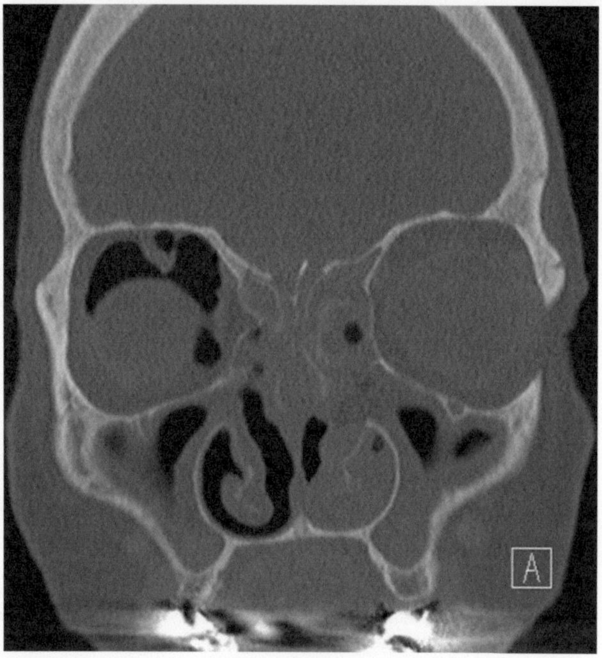

Fig. 7.2 Case 2. Computed tomography of postoperative patient complaining of diplopia

anesthesia and may have had positive pressure masking after extubation. This could have led air to track into the orbit, a complication not previously described.

Lessons Learned

More than 15% of the American population suffers from sinus disease, and approximately 350,000 sinus surgeries are done per year to address this disease process in the United States [1]. Despite the high prevalence of both the disease and its surgical management, the surgeon must remain vigilant for the myriad of complications possible, rather than fall complacent due to the "routine" nature of these procedures. Multiple retrospective database studies of cases done after the year 2000 have reported the rate of major complications of endoscopic sinus surgery at 0.36–1.0% [1, 2]. Major complications include, but are not limited to, hemorrhage, cerebrospinal fluid leak, meningitis, orbital hematoma, optic nerve injury, extraocular muscle injury, and lacrimal duct injury [2–4]. Reported rates of orbital complications of ESS vary from 0.07–0.66% [1, 2, 4], and a vast majority of these complications are due to iatrogenic exposed orbital fat, muscle injury, or hematoma.

The first case illustrates that surgeons should be careful with forceful irrigation in the case of extensive disease that may have thinned bony partitions. Additionally, it highlights that imaging may not reveal all of a patient's anatomic intricacies.

Knowledge and evaluation of anatomic landmarks intraoperatively are crucial to avoiding complications.

The second case demonstrates the importance of communication with the entire perioperative team. In a patient in whom there is a known bony dehiscence, it is best to warn our anesthesia colleagues so they may avoid positive pressure mask ventilation. Knowledge and careful consideration of all parts of the patient's perioperative management may lead to fewer complications.

While rare, orbital complications of ESS do occur at a rate of less than 1% and a vast majority of these involve hematomas and fat and muscle injury. Presented above are two rare but manageable complications. Otolaryngologists should be aware of potential complications and counsel patients preoperatively. Furthermore, they should be equipped to manage orbital complications of ESS, some of which may simply require observation and self-resolve.

References

1. Ramakrishnan VR, Kingdom TT, Nayak JV, Hwang PH, Orlandi RR. Nationwided incidence of major complications in endoscopic sinus surgery. Int Forum Allergy Rhinol. 2012;2:34–9.
2. Krings JG, Kallogjeri D, Wineland A, Nepple KG, Piccirillo JF, Getz AE. Complications of primary and revision functional endoscopic sinus surgery for chronic rhinosinusitis. Laryngoscope. 2014;124(4):838–45.
3. Stankiewicz JA, Lal D, Connor M, Welch K. Complications in endoscopic sinus surgery for chronic rhinosinusitis: a 25-year experience. Laryngoscope. 2011;121:2684–701.
4. Seredyka-Burduk M, Burdu PK, Wierzchowska M, Kaluzny B, Malukiewicz G. Ophthalmic complications of endoscopic sinus surgery. Braz J Otorhinolaryngol. 2017;83(3):318–23.

Chapter 8
Brown Syndrome Following Endoscopic Modified Lothrop Procedure

Rodolfo Prestinary and Roy Casiano

Clinical Pearls

1. Brown syndrome from an iatrogenic cause can happen after endoscopic sinus surgery.
2. The proximity of the frontal infundibulum to the trochlear fossa needs to be taken into account when using power instrumentation or monopolar suction cautery.
3. When drilling is required in the lateral frontal infundibulum and adjacent medial orbital roof, the surgeon should consider a diamond burr rather than a cutting burr, and if periorbita is exposed, a bipolar suction and cottonoids soaked in adrenalin for hemostasis.

Case Presentation

A 41-year-old female with a history of allergic fungal rhinosinusitis underwent endoscopic sinus surgery (ESS) 2 years prior. A bilateral total ethmoidectomy, sphenoid, maxillary, and Draf IIb frontal sinusotomies were performed. Over the course of 2 years, the patient experienced progressive symptoms of frontal pressure and discolored thick secretions. On nasal endoscopy there was significant crusting and allergic mucin bilaterally requiring repeated debridements. The mucin was predominantly observed from the anterior ethmoid cavity and frontal recess area. There were also moderate polypoid changes throughout her sinus cavities. A non-contrast CT scan was performed revealing moderate mucoperiosteal thickening of her frontal and ethmoid sinuses with osteoneogenesis (Fig. 8.1). After failing multiple

R. Prestinary (✉) · R. Casiano
Department of Otolaryngology, University of Miami, Miami, FL, USA
e-mail: rodolfo.prestinarye@jhsmiami.org

R. K. Chandra, K. C. Welch (eds.), *Lessons Learned from Rhinologic Procedure Complications*, https://doi.org/10.1007/978-3-030-75323-8_8

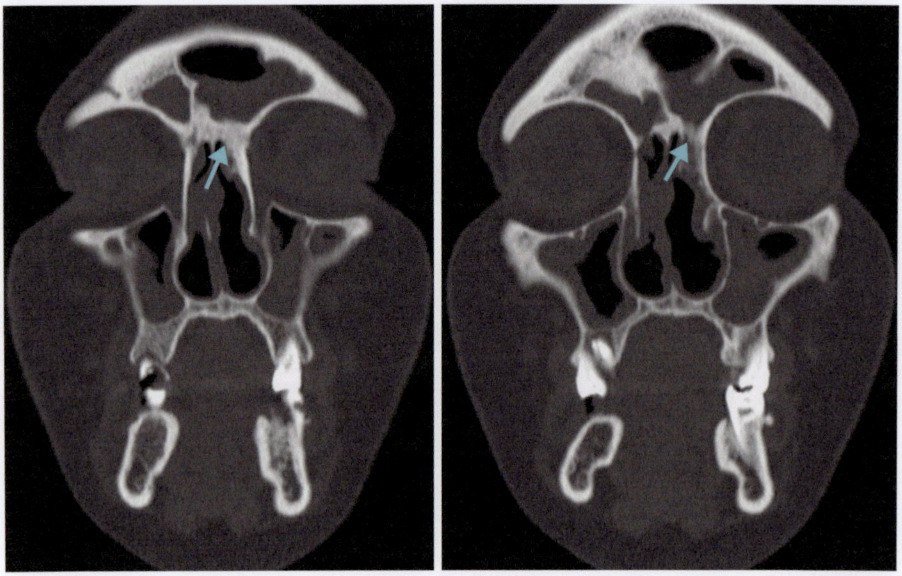

Fig. 8.1 Preoperative coronal and axial CT scan showing anterior ethmoid and frontal infundibular opacification with osteoneogenesis of the frontal infundibulum (arrow)

attempts at maximum medical therapy including high-volume irrigations, oral and topical corticosteroids (including budesonide), and culture-directed topical and oral antibiotics, revision surgery was advised. An extended sphenoidotomy, mega-maxillary antrostomies, and extended frontal sinusotomy (Draf III or modified Lothrop procedure) were performed to facilitate long-term debridements as well as the use of topical anti-inflammatory and antimicrobial management of the respective sinus cavities. During the surgery, dense allergic mucin, osteoneogenesis, and polypoid mucosa were present in all the sinuses. During the modified Lothrop portion of the surgery, the left anterosuperior orbital periosteum, in the area of the trochlea, was thinned with a cutting burr resulting in an inadvertent perirobita laceration. Mild bleeding in the tiny rent of torn periorbita was controlled with suction cautery followed by a topical 1:1000 adrenaline-soaked neurosurgical cottonoid.

Immediately postoperatively, in the recovery room, the patient complained of persistent diplopia, which was initially thought to be due to acute inflammation and edema from the bony drill-out. High-dose corticosteroids and antibiotics were administered. An ophthalmology evaluation was performed showing 20/25 vision bilaterally, and an abnormal traction test. The patient exhibited exotropia and hypotropia of the left eye with constant diplopia in all positions of gaze. A left-side hypotropia with downshoot was documented on left-eye adduction (Fig. 8.2). The exam characteristics were initially thought to be consistent with inferior rectus entrapment (which was not evident on CT), but later revised to be consistent with an acquired Brown syndrome on the left. A CT scan was performed (Fig. 8.3), showing

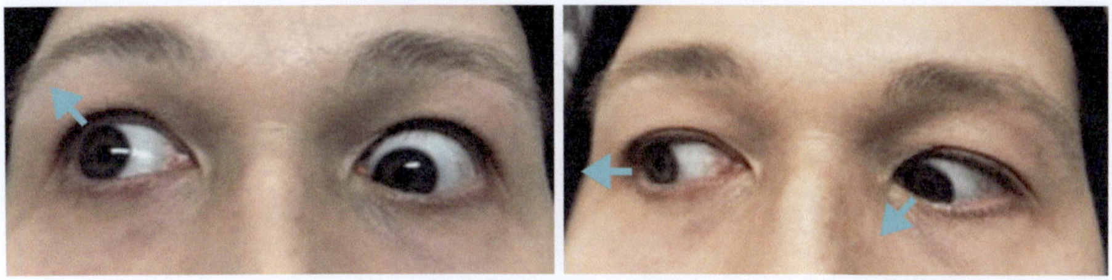

Fig. 8.2 Right superolateral gaze with limited superomedial adduction of the left eye (left image). Right lateral gaze with limited superomedial adduction of the left eye (right image)

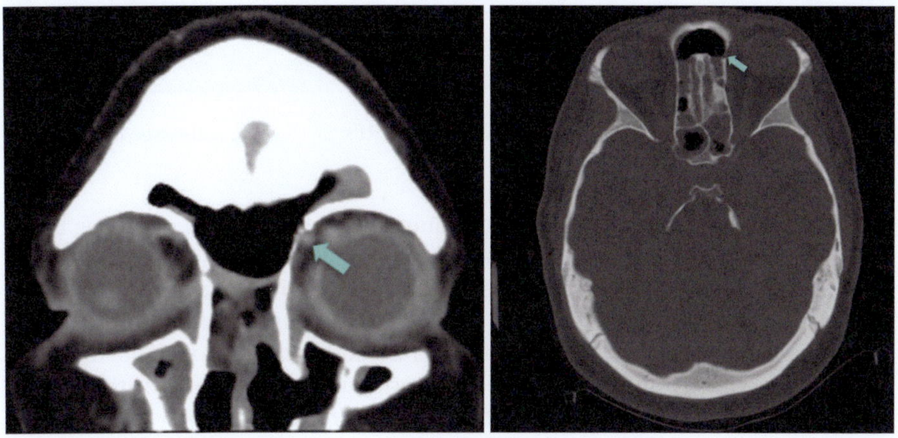

Fig. 8.3 Coronal (left) and axial (right) postoperative CT scan showing soft-tissue inflammation around the trochlear area (arrow) with bony dehiscence

a bony dehiscence near the left trochlear area. An MRI scan (Fig. 8.4) showed post-surgical changes noted around the soft tissues of the orbit around the trochlea.

At last follow-up (2 years after her ESS) she remains with slight diplopia on neutral gaze. Ophthalmology discussed treatment options and observation with no strabismus surgery was recommended. She remains free of sinus disease without any polypoid changes, crusts, or mucin production, on saline volume irrigations with budesonide.

Root Cause Analysis

Brown syndrome, also known as superior oblique tendon sheath syndrome, is rare. Most cases that have been reported are secondary to non-endoscopic (external) approaches to the ethmoid or frontal sinuses, mainly using a Lynch-type of

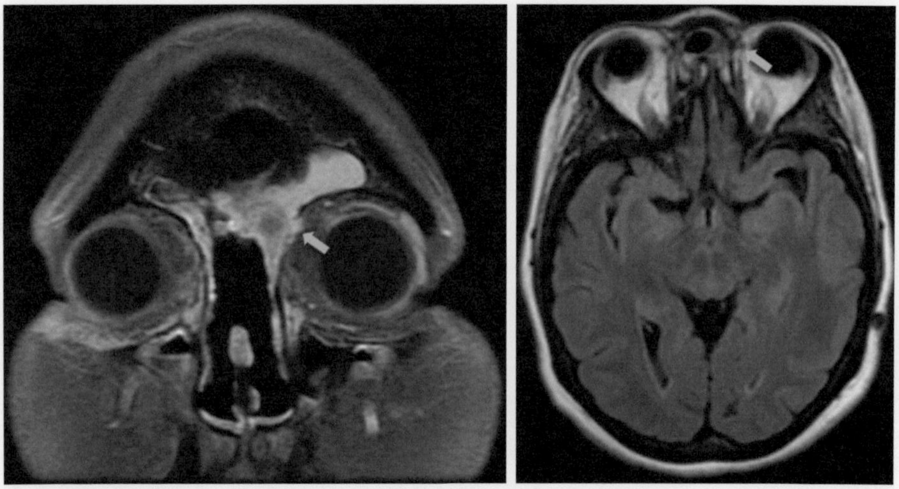

Fig. 8.4 Coronal (left) and axial (right) postoperative MRI scan showing soft-tissue inflammation around the trochlear area (arrow)

incision. Herein we illustrate a case of acquired Brown syndrome occurring under plausible but highly unexpected conditions, highlighting the surgeon's need for constant vigilance for unfathomable circumstances. Intraoperative video was reviewed, which revealed a failure to identify the area in the lateral frontal infundibulum corresponding to the trochlear fossa intraorbitally. Although the orbit was palpated periodically during the procedure, periorbita exposure in this area was not recognized, and drilling continued with a cutting burr, resulting in laceration of the periorbita and subsequent trochlear tendon injury. Aggressive use of cutting burrs and/or monopolar cautery in the area of the trochlear fossa subsequently resulted in a trauma to the trochlear fossa, although scans did not reveal any actual muscle or tendon injury.

Lessons Learned

According to Bartley et al., trochlear damage could occur with prolonged traction of the soft tissue near the trochlea with edema of the vascular sheath, fibrosis, and hypomotility of the tendon sheath [1]. In this case, as previously reported in the literature on one case, widening of the frontal infundibulum anterosuperiorly, can expose the periorbita in the area of the trochlea. A better alternative would have been to use a diamond burr when working in this area, with periodic palpation of the eye, to identified dehiscent periosteum or more importantly orbital fat or muscle. Even if the periorbita is preserved, one should not use monopolar cautery in this area if bleeding is encountered. Cottonoids soaked in 1:1000 adrenaline should suffice.

The trochlea is a cartilaginous pulley structure located in the nasal aspect of the frontal bone through which passes the tendon of the superior oblique muscle. Its main function is to provide a pulley system for the abduction, depression, and internal rotation of the eye. The trochlear anatomical location and relationship within the orbit is illustrated on Fig. 8.5. This cartilaginous structure is located in the trochlear fossa, which is a depression found in the anteromedial aspect of the orbit. The medial bony wall of the fossa corresponds with the lateral bone wall of the area of the anterolateral frontal infundibulum as seen endoscopically. The superior oblique muscle origin is above the annulus of Zinn and travels against the superiomedial orbital wall with its chord-like tendon passing through the trochlea and inserting in the superotemporal quadrant of the sclera [2].The proximity of the trochlear fossa in the anteromedial aspect of the orbit to the frontal sinus infundibulum is appreciated in Fig. 8.6. MRI imaging can also be used to visualize the trochlear tendon and superior oblique muscle (Fig. 8.7) [3].

Orbital muscle complications following ESS have being reported since endoscopic surgery was described in the 1980s. Brown syndrome is a rare cause of strabismus, characterized by limited elevation of the affected eye with an incidence of 1 in 450–500 strabismus cases [2]. It was first described by an American ophthalmologist, Harold W. Brown, who initially described it as superior oblique tendon sheath syndrome. Brown syndrome can be congenital or acquired. Congenital abnormalities have been described, such as an inelastic muscle or tendon, and abnormal orbital adhesions with tendon anomalies. Acquired Brown syndrome may be caused by trauma, such as in a motor vehicle accident or due to sports injuries. It may also occur with iatrogenic injury secondary to frontal sinus surgery [1], during blepharoplasty [4], or inflammatory causes secondary to systemic diseases such as systemic lupus erythematosus [5]. Brown syndrome can also be secondary to chronic sinus disease and throchleitis.

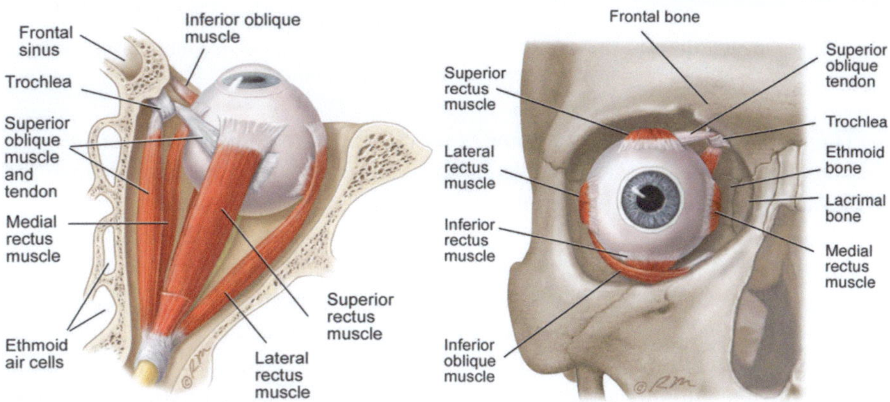

Fig. 8.5 Axial and coronal illustrations of the orbit. The relationship between the trochlear tendon and the frontal bone is appreciated

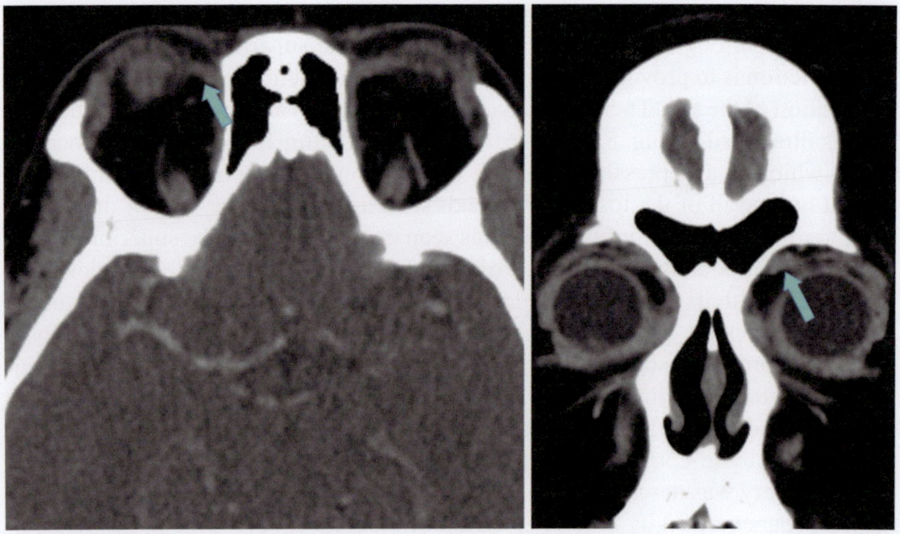

Fig. 8.6 Axial and coronal CT scans illustrating the proximity of the trochlear tendon with the frontal sinus (arrow)

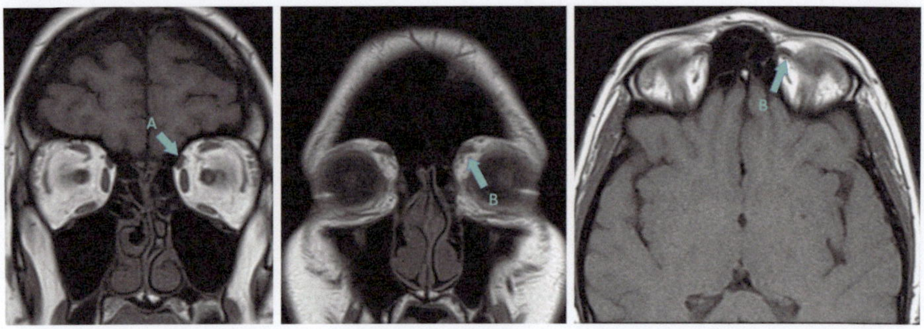

Fig. 8.7 Axial and coronal MRI images documenting the superior oblique muscle and trochlear tendon (arrows). Superior oblique muscle (**a**) and trochlear tendon (**b**)

The diagnosis of Brown syndrome is based on the patient's history and clinical findings. The patient may report a variety of symptoms, which may include inability to elevate the eye in adduction, diplopia, lengthening of the palpebral fissure, abnormal head position, and pain in the superior and inner angle of the orbit, secondary to supratrochlear nerve irritation, mainly in cases of inflammatory or posttraumatic conditions. On examination, the patient can present with limited elevation in adduction and a positive forced duction for restricted elevation in adduction. An anomalous head posture and ipsilateral hypotonia in primary position can also be seen. When Brown syndrome is caused by inflammatory etiologies, trochlear tenderness with a palpable click may be present that can sometime be heard by the patient on eye movement.

In acquired cases of Brown syndrome, a high-resolution MRI can define in great detail the pathological anatomical abnormalities causing Brown syndrome. The MRI findings include the presence of traumatic or iatrogenic scarring, avulsion of the trochlea, a cyst in the superior oblique tendon, an inferior displacement of the lateral rectus pulley, and/or fibrous restrictive bands extending from the trochlea to the globe [6]. It should be noted that orbital floor fractures may also trap the orbital tissue in such a way as to simulate Brown syndrome.

Most cases reported in the literature are rare and preceded the endoscopic sinus surgery (ESS) era, using external approaches to the ethmoid or frontal sinus through a Lynch-type incision in most cases. There has only been one case of Brown syndrome in the endoscopic era. Similar to the illustrated case, the authors describe an injury secondary to orbital periosteum damage with power instrumentation during an extended frontal sinusotomy (modified Lothrop) for access to repair a CSF leak [7]. On this case, the periorbita was drawn into the suction portion of the drill near the area of the superior oblique muscle. They concluded that the introduction of new powered tools for endoscopic surgery may necessitate care during dissection to avoid orbital complications [7].

References

1. Bartley J, Eagleton N, Rosser P, Al-Ali S. Superior oblique muscle palsy after frontal sinus mini-trephine. Am J Otolaryngol. 2012;33(1):181–3.
2. Abdelhady A, Patel B, Motlagh M, Al Aboud D. Anatomy, head and neck, eye superior oblique muscle. In: StatPearls [Internet] (2020). https://www.ncbi.nlm.nih.gov/books/NBK537152/. Accessed 10 Apr 2020.
3. Bhola R. Acute acquired brown syndrome: In: EyeRounds.org: Acute Acquired Brown Syndrome: 38 year-old Male with Ethmoidal Sinus Mucocele. https://webeye.ophth.uiowa.edu/eyeforum/cases/50-Acquired-Brown-Syndrome-Ethmoid-Mucocele.htm (2005). Accessed 15 Mar 2020.
4. Levine MR, Boynton J, Tenzel RR, Miller GR. Complications of blepharoplasty. Ophthalmic Surg. 1975;6:47–53.
5. Whitefield L, Isenberg DA, Brazier DJ, Forbes J. Acquired Brown's syndrome in systemic lupus erythematosus. Br J Rheumatol. 1995;34:1092–4.
6. Bhola R, Rosenbaum AL, Ortube M, Demer JL. High resolution MRI demonstrates varied anatomic abnormalities in Brown's syndrome. J AAPOS. 2005;9(1):438–48.
7. Leibovitch I, Wormald PJ, Crompton J, Selva D. Iatrogenic Brown's syndrome during EndoscopicSinus surgery with powered instruments. Otolaryngol Head Neck Surg. 2005;133:300–1.

References

Part II
The Skull Base

Chapter 9
Ethmoid CSF Cerebrospinal Fluid Leak

Tran B. Locke and Nithin D. Adappa

Clinical Pearls

1. Major complications of endoscopic sinus surgery (ESS) such as intracranial injury and cerebrospinal fluid (CSF) leaks still occur and may be related to failure to appreciate surgical anatomy and poor visualization during surgery.
2. Repair of iatrogenic CSF leaks can be performed using any combination of grafting material, tissue sealants, or autologous tissue. For referred cases, the use of intrathecal injection of diluted 10% fluorescein can help identify the location of the CSF leak or skull base defect.
3. If reconstruction of CSF leaks is not part of routine otolaryngology practice, consideration for referral is suggested so as to minimize risk of any further complications.

Case Presentation

A 29-year-old male underwent bilateral endoscopic sinus surgery with septoplasty that was complicated by an intraoperative CSF leak. The leak was repaired by the primary otolaryngologist at the time of injury using septal cartilage and bone with fibrin glue. Postoperative imaging demonstrated migration of a 5 mm plate of bone from the right fovea ethmoidalis defect into the inferior frontal lobe (Fig. 9.1).

T. B. Locke
Department of Otolaryngology – Head and Neck Surgery, Baylor College of Medicine, Houston, TX, USA

N. D. Adappa (✉)
Department of Otorhinolaryngology - Head and Neck Surgery, University of Pennsylvania, Philadelphia, PA, USA
e-mail: Nithin.adappa@pennmedicine.upenn.edu

R. K. Chandra, K. C. Welch (eds.), *Lessons Learned from Rhinologic Procedure Complications*, https://doi.org/10.1007/978-3-030-75323-8_9

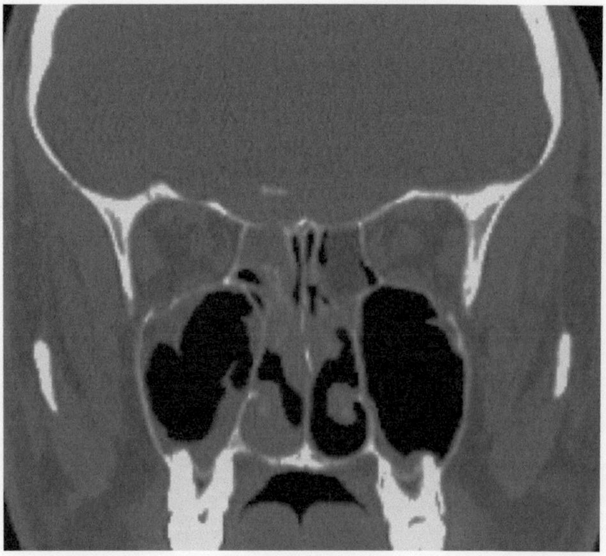

Fig. 9.1 Coronal CT demonstrating migrated bone graft from initially attempted CSF leak closure

Patient was transferred to us for care. On admission, he was noted to have unilateral clear rhinorrhea. Given the concern for an active CSF leak, the decision was made to proceed to the OR for exploration of the traumatic site and repair of the skull base defect.

The frontal recess was dissected to expose the ethmoid skull base defect. Stereotactic navigation was used to confirm the location of the leak (Fig. 9.2). Various pieces of cartilage and bony fragments were removed from the frontal lobe. A 3 × 3 mm dural tear was exposed and bipolar cautery was used to control bleeding along the rim of the tear. A multilayer repair using dural matrix was placed into the dura and into the epidural space to cover the length of the bony defect followed by fibrin glue. The surrounding nasal mucosa around the bony defect was removed, and a piece of middle turbinate bone graft was cut to size and used as an inlay graft to create appropriate closure and support in the area. A nasoseptal flap was raised and then rotated into position over the skull base defect, fibrin glue applied, and nasal packing placed (Fig. 9.3). Postoperatively, the patient was placed on bedrest for 48 h. Postoperative imaging showed repair of the defect with overlying nasoseptal flap (Fig. 9.4). Fortunately, the patient had no intracranial injury or neurologic sequela but, in this instance, while the initial CSF leak occurred, additional intracranial injury could have occurred due to displacement of bone graft in intracranial space.

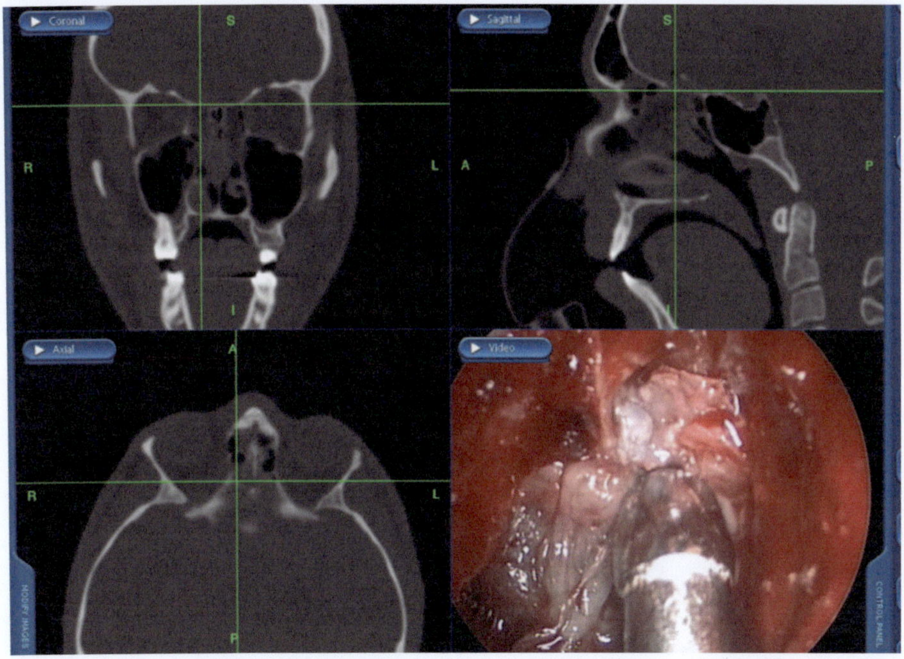

Fig. 9.2 Use of stereotactic image-guided navigation to confirm site of leak

Root Cause Analysis

Avoidance of Intraoperative CSF Leaks

Endoscopic sinus surgery (ESS) is effective at addressing medically recalcitrant sinus disease. The addition of stereotactic image-guided navigation and advances in surgical techniques have revolutionized the procedure, potentially allowing surgeons to perform more thorough dissection while minimizing risks to surrounding structures. Despite these advances, surgeons must not develop a false sense of security as complications still occur. Iatrogenic injury during endoscopic sinus surgery accounts for 16% of anterior skull base CSF leaks with the most common site of injury being the cribriform plate or fovea ethmoidalis (80%) and less commonly the frontal sinus (8%) and sphenoid sinus (4%) [1]. Failure to appreciate anatomic relationships and asymmetry, poor visualization due to bleeding, and previous surgery are factors that may lead to CSF leak [2].

Several steps can be taken to prevent iatrogenic injury to the skull base. Preoperative considerations include thorough review of the patient's anatomy using the interactive triplanar (or perhaps three-dimensional) software associated with image-guided navigation system, selection of appropriate instrumentation, and understanding the patient's comorbidities.

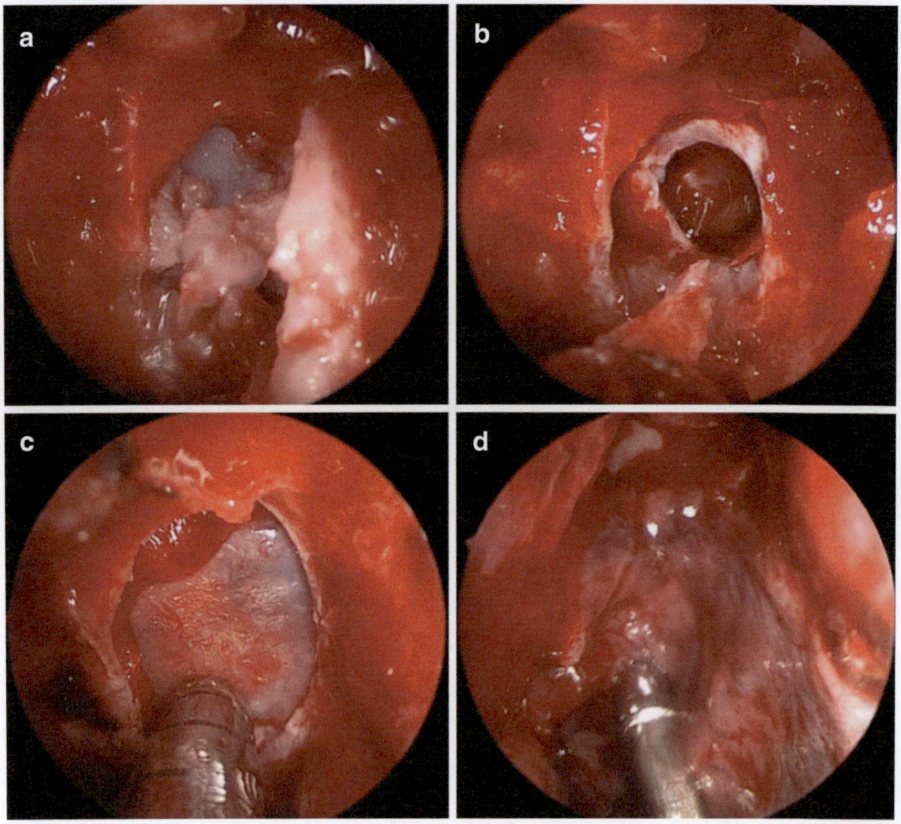

Fig. 9.3 Intraoperative repair of skull base defect. (**a**) Fragments of cartilage removed form defect. (**b**) Dural defect exposed and surrounding area prepared. (**c**) Middle turbinate bone utilized as inlay graft. (**d**) Nasoseptal flap onlay positioned over defect

Understanding the skull base anatomy is crucial in sinus surgery. All patients undergoing endoscopic sinus surgery should have a thin-slice (1–3 mm) computed tomography (CT) scan of sinus for image-guided navigation to help understand the relationship between the paranasal sinuses and anterior skull base. The CT scan can highlight certain areas of interest which are high risk for iatrogenic injury, such as asymmetry of the skull base or areas of bony thinning or dehiscence. For instance, the coronal cuts can reveal the length of the lateral cribriform lamella (Keros classification), ratio of maxillary-to-ethmoid height, and thickness of the anterior skull base. Sagittal images help evaluate the slope of the skull base, anterior-posterior diameter of the frontal recess, and frontal sinus cells [3, 4].

- The Keros classification describes the length of the lateral cribriform lamella as it relates to the fovea ethmoidalis. There are three grades of depth: type 1 (1–3 mm), type II (4–7 mm), and type III (8–16 mm). Risk for intracranial injury

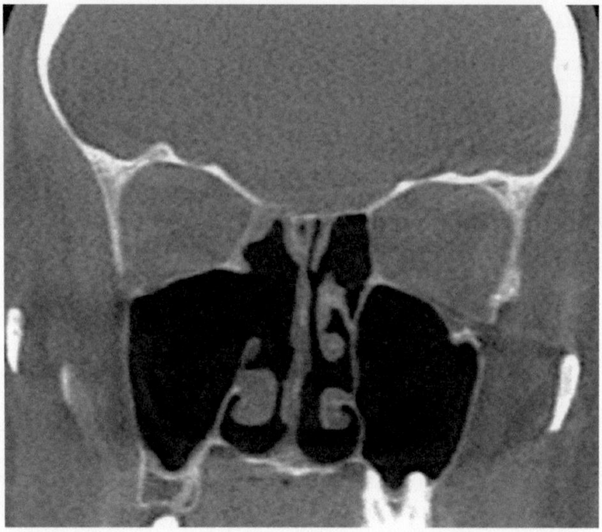

Fig. 9.4 Coronal CT demonstrating repair of previous skull base defect and CSF leak

is positively correlated with higher Keros classification yielding a higher risk of iatrogenic injury.

- The maxillary-to-ethmoid height can be used to guide dissection through the posterior ethmoid cells. The greater the ratio, the higher is the risk for iatrogenic injury to the anterior skull base.
- Similarly, a steeper slope to the skull base can predispose to injury, particularly around the medial posterior ethmoid cells.

It is crucial to ensure that all equipment is functioning properly prior to the start of the case. The use of image-guided navigation and appropriate sinus instrumentation can assist with a thorough intraoperative dissection of the paranasal sinuses. However, a poorly calibrated navigation system or lack of adequate sinus instruments can mislead a surgeon into a dangerous situation. In addition, hemostasis is critical to maintaining good visualization of the operative field. Consideration should be given to total intravenous anesthesia and the use of topical vasoconstriction to prevent obscuration of the surgical bed and landmarks (the authors use 1:1000 epinephrine-soaked pledgets).

Certain patient factors, such as the presence of sinonasal tumors, previous endoscopic sinus surgery, bleeding, or nasal polyps can distort the sinus anatomy and relationship between landmarks [2]. In addition, comorbidities such as benign intracranial hypertension, high body-mass index, mucoceles, or allergic fungal sinusitis can thin the bone of the anterior skull base [5]. The surgeon should take note of these risk factors and cross correlate it with the patient's CT scan.

Management of Intraoperative CSF Leaks

Injuries to the skull base can still happen despite thorough knowledge of the patient's anatomy, use of stereotactic image-guided navigation, and safe surgical techniques. When an intraoperative leak occurs, the surgeon should stop, reorient oneself, and utilize the stereotactic imaging to localize the site of leak. In addition, identification of an intraoperative CSF leak can be a stressful event and often leads a surgeon who may not perform a high volume of repairs to cause further complications.

There are three goals after identification of the leak [4]:

1. Ensuring safe and successful closure of the leak
2. Preserving sinus function
3. Prevention of postoperative complications

When concern for skull base injury has occurred, we recommend placing a thrombin-soaked or plain pledget over the area to help with hemostasis, putting the procedure on pause, and re-reviewing the CT scan. This will often give the surgeon time to regain his/her composure. Once the defect is found, the surrounding site should be prepared. The adjacent sinuses and all residual partitions should be taken down such that a flat surface surrounding the defect is achieved (Fig. 9.3b) with a minimum rim of 2–3 mm. The mucosa adjacent to the defect should be cauterized with bipolar cautery on low setting and gently stripped away. Next, the defect size should be measured. The size of the defect can be used to dictate the type of repair required for success [2, 4, 5]:

- Defects less than 2 mm will heal via osteoneogenesis and soft-tissue fibrosis. These small defects can be repaired using an overlay free mucosal graft from the middle turbinate, nasal floor, or septum. Alternatively, use of a synthetic graft can be considered if no autologous option is available.
- Defects 2–6 mm in size can be repaired with a composite graft using middle turbinate or septal bone as an underlay graft and free mucosa as an overlay graft.
- Defects greater than 6 mm can be closed in a multilayer fashion with underlay bone graft (septum or turbinate) and an overlay vascularized nasoseptal flap or free mucosal graft (Fig. 9.3c, d). The choice of a free mucosal graft or vascularized pedicle flap is contingent on the defect location and velocity of CSF flow.

The repairs described above are presented in increasing complexity. To ensure success, all materials should be prepared and ready for use prior to initiating closure of the intracranial defect. Once the defect site is cleared, sequential repair is performed in a meticulous and methodical fashion. The grafts and/or pedicled flap are maneuvered and positioned into place. Fibrin sealant is then applied between placement of the inlay and onlay grafts. Gentle packing with Vaseline gauze and frontal sinus stents can be used to hold the repair material in place. The use of nasal trumpets to help bolster the repair and divert airflow into the nasopharynx should be considered for large anterior skull base defects.

Due to the proximity of the cribriform plate, care should be exercised during repair of ethmoid CSF leaks to avoid inadvertent worsening of the defect or further complications. Repair should be attempted based on the surgeon's experience and comfort level. If the surgeon is unable to repair the defect, hemostasis should be obtained, the nasal cavity gently packed, and the patient transferred to a rhinologist [4]. CT angiography head should be performed to ensure no hematoma or vascular injury has occurred. Neurosurgery consultation should be considered for further assessment of intracranial injury.

Secondary CSF leak repair can be difficult due to postoperative edema and scarring. While imaging can help with localization, it may be difficult to identify the site in a postoperative patient. In these circumstances, one option for identification of a leak site is via intraoperative blue light endoscopy after intrathecal fluorescein injection. The use of intrathecal fluorescein is not FDA approved and informed consent should be obtained, with the inclusion of neurological complications such as headaches, seizures, and cranial nerve deficits. The recommended dose within the literature is 0.1 ml of 10% fluorescein in 10 mL of CSF injected over a 10-min period [5–7].

While careful intraoperative repair is important, postoperative considerations are equally critical in optimizing the success of an ethmoid CSF leak repair. For instance, efforts should be made to decrease intracranial pressure with deep extubation and avoidance of positive airway pressure. All patients should be placed on bed rest for approximately 24–48 h depending on the severity of the CSF leak. Antiemetics and stool softeners should be scheduled in the immediate postoperative period to avoid accidental increases in pressure on the repair site. The patient should also be advised to avoid blowing their nose or Valsalva maneuvers for the aforementioned reason. Packing should be left in place for at least several days to facilitate healing. Intravenous and subsequent oral antibiotics that cross the blood brain barrier should be administered as prophylaxis.

Lessons Learned

Despite advances in imaging and stereotactic technology, endoscopic instrumentation, and anatomic understanding, iatrogenic CSF leak remains a viable concern during endoscopic sinus surgery. Repair of anterior fossa CSF leaks can be done endoscopically with a success rate of 90–94% [5, 8]. However, failure to recognize the situation, lack of proper equipment, or inexperience may lead to more complications during the repair of a CSF leak. It is of paramount importance that while a single complication has occurred during surgery, avoidance of any further complications is critical. If the defect cannot be identified or if the surgeon is unable to adequately repair the defect, hemostasis should be achieved and the nasal cavity gently packed. In addition, the patient should receive perioperative antibiotics that cross the blood brain barrier, a deep extubation to avoid increases in intracranial pressure, and a CT head (or a CT angiography if concerned for vascular injury that can occur if a microdebrider has entered the intracranial space). Ultimately, once stabilized and clinically safe, the patient should be transferred to a local rhinologist or skull base surgeon for continuation of care.

References

1. Le C, Strong EB, Luu Q. Management of anterior skull base cerebrospinal fluid leaks. J Neurol Surg Part B Skull Base. 2016;77(5):404–11.
2. Hegazy HM, Carrau RL, Snyderman CH, Kassam A, Zweig J. Transnasal endoscopic repair of cerebrospinal fluid rhinorrhea: a meta-analysis. Laryngoscope. 2000;110(7):1166–72.
3. Heaton CM, Goldberg AN, Pletcher SD, Glastonbury CM. Sinus anatomy associated with inadvertent cerebrospinal fluid leak during functional endoscopic sinus surgery. Laryngoscope. 2012;122(7):1446–9.
4. Welch KC, Palmer JN. Intraoperative emergencies during endoscopic sinus surgery: CSF leak and orbital hematoma. Otolaryngol Clin N Am. 2008;41(3):581–96. ix–x
5. Bedrosian JC, Anand VK, Schwartz TH. The endoscopic endonasal approach to repair of iatrogenic and noniatrogenic cerebrospinal fluid leaks and encephaloceles of the anterior cranial fossa. World Neurosurg. 2014;82(6 Suppl):S86–94.
6. Banks CA, Palmer JN, Chiu AG, O'Malley BW Jr, Woodworth BA, Kennedy DW. Endoscopic closure of CSF rhinorrhea: 193 cases over 21 years. Otolaryngol Head Neck Surg. 2009;140(6):826–33.
7. Placantonakis DG, Tabaee A, Anand VK, Hiltzik D, Schwartz TH. Safety of low-dose intrathecal fluorescein in endoscopic cranial base surgery. Neurosurgery. 2007;61(3 Suppl):161–5. discussion 5–6
8. Konuthula N, Khan MN, Del Signore A, Govindaraj S, Shrivastava R, Iloreta AM. A systematic review of secondary cerebrospinal fluid leaks. Am J Rhinol Allergy. 2017;31(6):48–56.

Chapter 10
Sphenoid Cerebrospinal Fluid Leak

Jessica W. Grayson and Bradford A. Woodworth

Clinical Pearls

1. Drawing expertise from colleagues in other specialties allows a collaborative approach in the care of the complex sphenoid CSF leak patient.
2. Infections are unlikely to clear in the presence of a foreign body, despite the use of broad-spectrum antibiotics.
3. Post-radiation defects of the sphenoid, particularly with exposed large caliber vessels, require vascularized tissue coverage and multiple coverage options should be considered.

Case Presentation

A 58-year-old female with a history of acromegaly secondary to pituitary tumor underwent endoscopic trans-sphenoidal resection in 2007 (followed by gamma knife therapy in 2008 for residual tumor). She had six subsequent endoscopic sinus surgeries (ESS) for a persistent *Pseudomonas aeruginosa* infection of the sphenoid sinuses. In 2018, she developed several recurrent episodes of large-volume epistaxis and was found to have a left carotid pseudoaneurysm. An interventional radiologist performed endovascular coiling, but she continued to have life-threatening episodes

Supplementary Information The online version of this chapter (https://doi.org/10.1007/978-3-030-75323-8_10) contains supplementary material, which is available to authorized users.

J. W. Grayson (✉) · B. A. Woodworth
Department of Otolaryngology Head and Neck Surgery, University of Alabama Birmingham, Birmingham, AL, USA
e-mail: jgrayson@uabmc.edu

R. K. Chandra, K. C. Welch (eds.), *Lessons Learned from Rhinologic Procedure Complications*, https://doi.org/10.1007/978-3-030-75323-8_10

of epistaxis. She also developed a clear watery rhinorrhea with head tilt. Following another large-volume bleed, her primary otolaryngologist brought her to the operating room for epistaxis control, identified a skull base defect and CSF leak (Beta 2 transferrin positive), and subsequently referred her for further management (Fig. 10.1). On endoscopy, she was noted to have a large septal defect, exposed ICA coils in the sphenoid sinus, purulence pooling at the base of the sinus in the presence of necrotic bone, and a 1 cm skull base defect with pulsatile clear fluid (Fig. 10.2). The sinus was cultured and returned ciprofloxacin-resistant *Pseudomonas aeruginosa*.

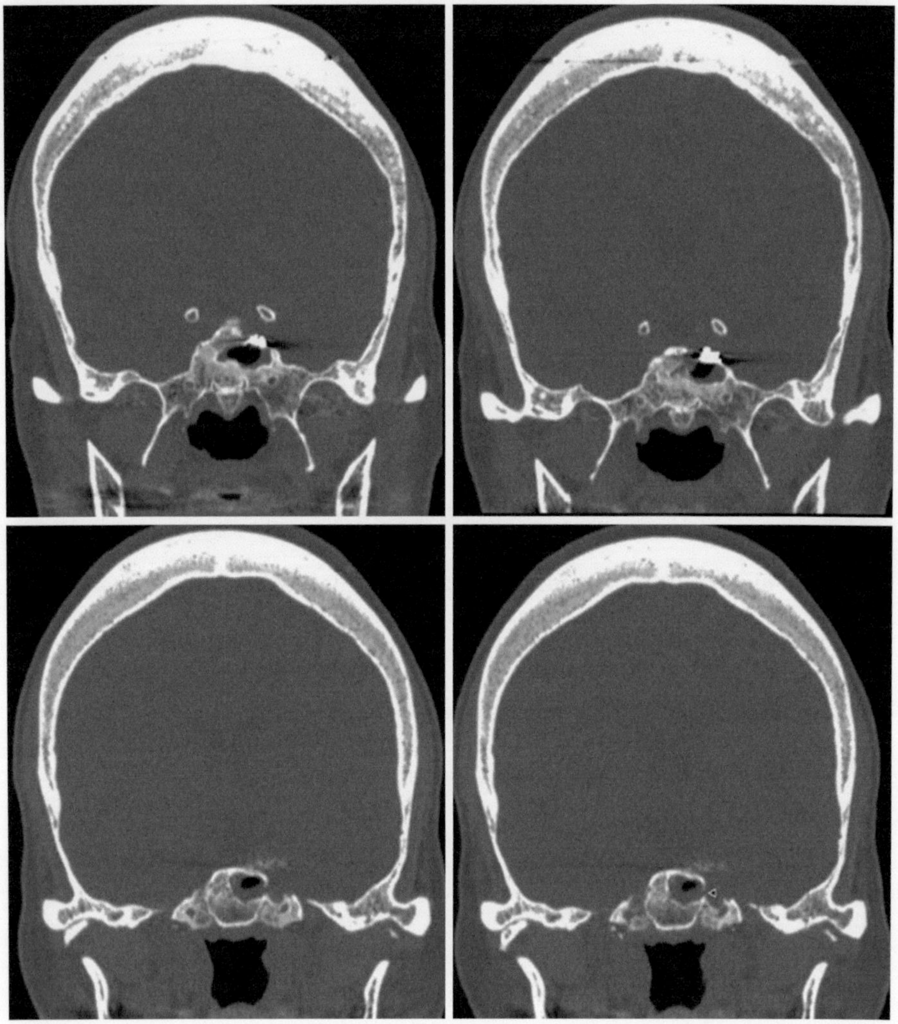

Fig. 10.1 Coronal computed tomography (CT) showing carotid coils as a hyperintense foreign body in the sphenoid and evidence of a skull base defect

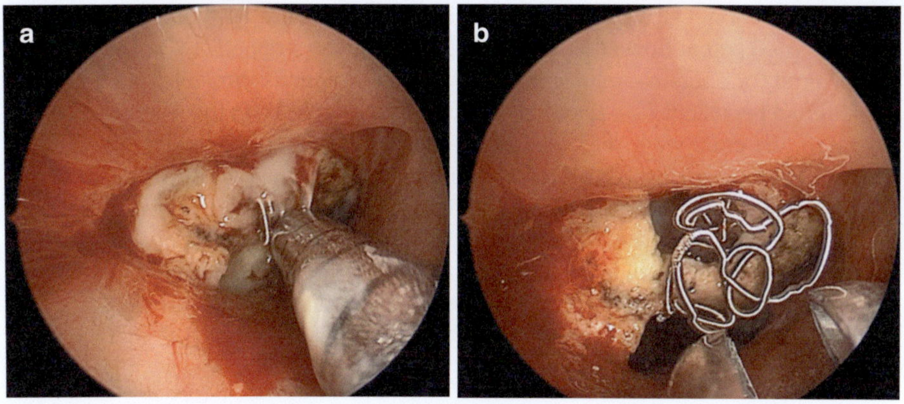

Fig. 10.2 Endoscopic view of the sphenoid sinus; (**a**) purulence noted in the sphenoid sinus; (**b**) carotid coils present in the sphenoid sinus with skull base defect noted

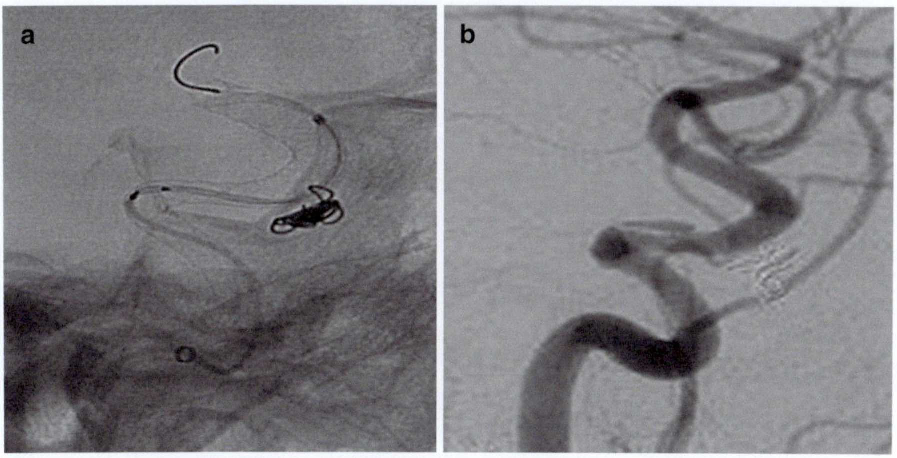

Fig. 10.3 Angiography of Pipeline™ internal carotid artery stent insertion (**a**) and patent flow at 3 months just prior to surgery (**b**)

Our neuro-interventional colleagues were consulted for analysis of the carotid circulation and possibility of carotid artery sacrifice. A balloon occlusion test (BOT) was performed and she was determined to have inadequate Circle of Willis blood flow to permit coiling of the internal carotid artery. Therefore, a Pipeline™ stent (Pipeline Flex Embolization Device, Medtronic, Jacksonville, FL) was inserted to bypass the coils and pseudoaneurysm (Fig. 10.3a). A delay in closure of the CSF leak was necessary due to the need for dual antiplatelet therapy for 3 months. The Infectious Disease team was consulted to treat the active *Pseudomonas* infection to decrease the risk of meningitis. A peripherally inserted central catheter was placed and chronic antibiotic therapy with cefepime was initiated. In the setting of a foreign body, the goal of therapy was to prevent meningitis, rather than completely clear the infection. Once the patient completed dual antiplatelet therapy and angiography showed patent flow at 3 months (Fig. 10.3b), she stopped the clopidogrel and was cleared for operative management. Despite continuous intravenous antibiotics, she still had persistent *Pseudomonas* infection at the site. With the pseudoaneurysm bypassed, the coils were removed under endoscopic guidance. Next, the necrotic, infected bone was drilled down to dura and the carotid artery. The skull base defect and CSF leak were repaired with a nasal floor flap designed to provide vascularized tissue in the absence of the septal mucosa (Video 10.1). The patient continued intravenous antibiotic therapy with cefepime for 3 months postoperatively. She is now 1-year post-treatment with no CSF leak or residual *Pseudomonas* infection.

Root Cause Analysis

This patient represents a complicated medical and surgical management scenario for a CSF leak in the sphenoid sinus. Root causes include (1) creation of a traumatic pseudoaneurysm, (2) radiation treatment, (3) inadequately treated *Pseudomonas* infection with osteomyelitis, and (4) repetitive trauma to the sphenoid bone from six endoscopic sinus surgeries. Complicating factors in management of this CSF leak include (1) sentinel bleeding from the carotid artery, (2) exposed endovascular coils, (3) quinolone-resistant *Pseudomonas* infection with risk of meningitis, (4) osteonecrosis/osteomyelitis, and (5) lack of septal mucosa for a robust nasoseptal flap option for reconstruction.

Lessons Learned

Patient care should occur at a tertiary hospital or a facility with appropriate medical and surgical personnel. Access to a neurosurgeon, neurosurgical ICU, neurointerventional radiologist (may be neurosurgeon or radiologist), infectious disease specialists, and skull base surgeon are essential in the care of this patient. Prioritizing the most urgent, life-threatening problems was critical to proper treatment. Due to multiple episodes of severe epistaxis from the carotid artery, this issue should take priority to avoid sudden death or anoxic brain injury. The two options to manage this level of bleeding are either carotid sacrifice or Pipeline™ stent bypass of the pseudoaneurysm. Sacrificing the carotid artery requires preoperative BOT to ensure that the patient has adequate Circle of Willis blood flow. However, ~10% of patients with adequate Circle of Willis flow on BOT will still suffer neurological sequelae from carotid sacrifice [1, 2]. If patients do not pass the BOT, a Pipeline™ stent is another option, but requires post-stenting antiplatelet therapy with aspirin and clopidogrel for 3 months.

A skull base defect and CSF leak in isolation does not typically require emergent management. However, the risk of meningitis increases in the presence of known infection and is the next priority following life-threatening carotid artery bleeding. Infections in the setting of foreign bodies are well known to be recalcitrant to medical management including intravenous antibiotic therapy. Biofilms can exist on the foreign body preventing the ability to clear the infection [3]. While removal of the foreign body is integral to definitive management of the infection, delayed surgical management due to dual antiplatelet therapy was required. The infectious disease specialists felt that cefepime would sufficiently suppress the infection to prevent meningitis.

Surgical management of a CSF leak requires preparation for multiple reconstructive options. While defects within the sphenoid sinus can be repaired with free mucosal grafts or allografts, the nasoseptal flap has become the workhorse for repair due to vascularized blood supply [4, 5]. In the current scenario, we felt vascularized tissue was necessary in the setting of osteoradionecrosis due to a decreased likelihood of repair success with nonvascularized approaches. Large caliber vessels and/or stents should also be covered with vascularized tissue. Given the previous loss of septal mucosa, a nasal floor flap was chosen to repair the defect. A porcine small intestine submucosal graft (Biodesign™, Cook Medical, Bloomington, IN) was placed first on the dura for additional support and over the portion of the right sphenoid sinus where there was insufficient flap coverage. The nasal floor flap is pedicled off the posterior septal artery, but also receives supply from greater palatine and superior labial arteries. The flap has a robust blood supply that can survive off any of one of these vessels' arterial supply [6]. The nasal floor flap is thinner than the nasoseptal flap, but can still be rotated and is pliable.

Postoperative supportive packing is paramount to the success of skull base repair and obviates the need for CSF diversion in many cases [7–10]. It is important to provide equal support across the defect to permit fibroblastic knitting of the tissue and ensure flap survival. Patients with prior radiation may have slowed healing, therefore adequate pressure to provide consistent contact to the repair and the underlying wound bed is crucial. In this patient, absorbable packing was placed as the first layer against the reconstruction. Ribbon gauze (1/2″) was then placed against the absorbable packing, which helps provide uniform distribution of pressure in this area. Cotton sponges in non-latex gloved finger were placed against the ribbon gauze packing at the intended location. Silastic splints were placed over the septal remnants to provide scaffolding support to the spacer. Packing was left in place for ~2–3 weeks.

Conclusion

Management of sphenoid CSF leaks is complicated in the setting of prior surgery and radiation. When there is additional complexity, it is critical to incorporate other subspecialists that can assist with treatment planning. Prioritizing the most emergent issues in the patient's care is also critical to successful outcomes.

References

1. Linskey ME, Jungreis CA, Yonas H, et al. Stroke risk after abrupt internal carotid artery sacrifice: accuracy of preoperative assessment with balloon test occlusion and stable xenon-enhanced CT. AJNR Am J Neuroradiol. 1994;15(5):829–43.
2. Mathis JM, Barr JD, Jungreis CA, et al. Temporary balloon test occlusion of the internal carotid artery: experience in 500 cases. AJNR Am J Neuroradiol. 1995;16(4):749–54.
3. Woodworth BA, Tamashiro E, Bhargave G, Cohen NA, Palmer JN. An in vitro model of Pseudomonas aeruginosa biofilms on viable airway epithelial cell monolayers. Am J Rhinol. 2008;22(3):235–8.
4. Alexander NS, Chaaban MR, Riley KO, Woodworth BA. Treatment strategies for lateral sphenoid sinus recess cerebrospinal fluid leaks. Arch Otolaryngol Head Neck Surg. 2012;138(5):471–8.
5. Chaaban MR, Illing E, Riley KO, Woodworth BA. Spontaneous cerebrospinal fluid leak repair: a five-year prospective evaluation. Laryngoscope. 2014;124(1):70–5.
6. Daraei P, Oyesiku NM, Patel ZM. The nasal floor pedicled flap: a novel technique for use in skull base reconstruction. Int Forum Allergy Rhinol. 2014;4(11):937–43.
7. Karnezis TT, Baker AB, Soler ZM, et al. Factors impacting cerebrospinal fluid leak rates in endoscopic sellar surgery. Int Forum Allergy Rhinol. 2016;6(11):1117–25.
8. Oakley GM, Orlandi RR, Woodworth BA, Batra PS, Alt JA. Management of cerebrospinal fluid rhinorrhea: an evidence-based review with recommendations. Int Forum Allergy Rhinol. 2016;6(1):17–24.
9. Illing E, Chaaban MR, Riley KO, Woodworth BA. Porcine small intestine submucosal graft for endoscopic skull base reconstruction. Int Forum Allergy Rhinol. 2013;3(11):928–32.
10. Wang EW, Zanation AM, Gardner PA, et al. ICAR: endoscopic skull-base surgery. Int Forum Allergy Rhinol. 2019;9(S3):S145–365.

Chapter 11
Cerebrospinal Fluid Leak and Pneumocephalus after FESS

Katie Phillips and Jayakar V. Nayak

Clinical Pearls

1. Understanding skull base anatomy – achieved through a combination of extensive analysis of imaging, cadaver, or stimulated dissections prior to surgery near skull base structures, and surgical experience – can help mitigate iatrogenic CSF leaks.
2. Careful review of anatomical variants (skull base slope and height, asymmetry, presence of certain air cells, bony dehiscences) prior to starting a FESS will alert surgeon to potential pitfalls.
3. If an iatrogenic CSF leak occurs during FESS, it is important to remain calm, recognizing this complication can be readily managed with good outcomes if proper procedures are followed to safely repair the defect.

Case Presentation

The patient is a 75-year-old male with a history of chronic rhinosinusitis for years, status post balloon sinuplasty with recurrence of sinonasal symptoms including chronic nasal congestion, recurrent sinusitis, facial pressure, frontal headaches, and post nasal drip which had been refractory to daily large-volume saline irrigations, topical corticosteroids and several courses of antibiotics and prednisone.

K. Phillips · J. V. Nayak (✉)
Department of Otolaryngology – Head and Neck Surgery, Stanford University School of Medicine, Stanford, CA, USA
e-mail: jnayak@stanford.edu

R. K. Chandra, K. C. Welch (eds.), *Lessons Learned from Rhinologic Procedure Complications*, https://doi.org/10.1007/978-3-030-75323-8_11

Functional endoscopic sinus surgery (FESS) was recommended and the patient underwent bilateral maxillary antrostomies, anterior ethmoidectomies, and frontal sinusotomies by an outside otolaryngologist. The patient called the office on postoperative day 1 (POD1) and noted left greater than right copious nasal discharge and conservative management was advised. On POD2, he then developed severe bitemporal headache, nausea, vomiting, and chills. Significantly, he reported his headache was exacerbated when standing and improved when lying down. He was advised to proceed to the emergency room, where postoperative imaging was consistent with extensive pneumocephalus and an unrecognized skull base bony defect at the junction of the fovea ethmoidalis and lateral lamella of the cribriform plate at the time of FESS (Fig. 11.1). Otolaryngology was consulted, and the patient was urgently taken to the operating suite for endoscopic repair of the skull base defect and CSF leak. A 2 mm × 2 mm defect was identified just superior to the anterior ethmoid artery, along the lateral lamella, without direct arterial injury (Fig. 11.2). The area around the defect was prepared by first ligating the anterior ethmoid artery using bipolar cautery, removing the surrounding remnant ethmoid cells along the skull base and then clearing a 3–4 mm circumference of mucosa around the defect. This skull base defect was repaired using a free mucosal overlay graft harvested from the contralateral nasal floor and secured with fibrin glue and resorbable nasal packing. Postoperatively, he noted improvement of his headache and he was subsequently discharged in stable condition and has been doing well at follow-up. He has smooth re-mucosalization of the left ethmoid skull base (Fig. 11.2c).

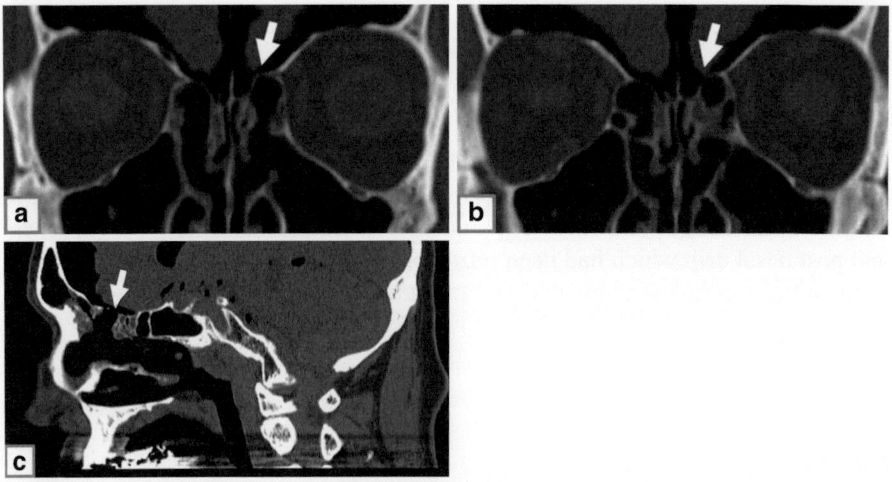

Fig. 11.1 (**a**, **b**) CT scan, coronal view of two sequential slices documenting left lateral lamella skull base defect noted via white arrow. (**c**) CT scan, sagittal view, with significant pneumocephalus noted and skull base defect noted via white arrow

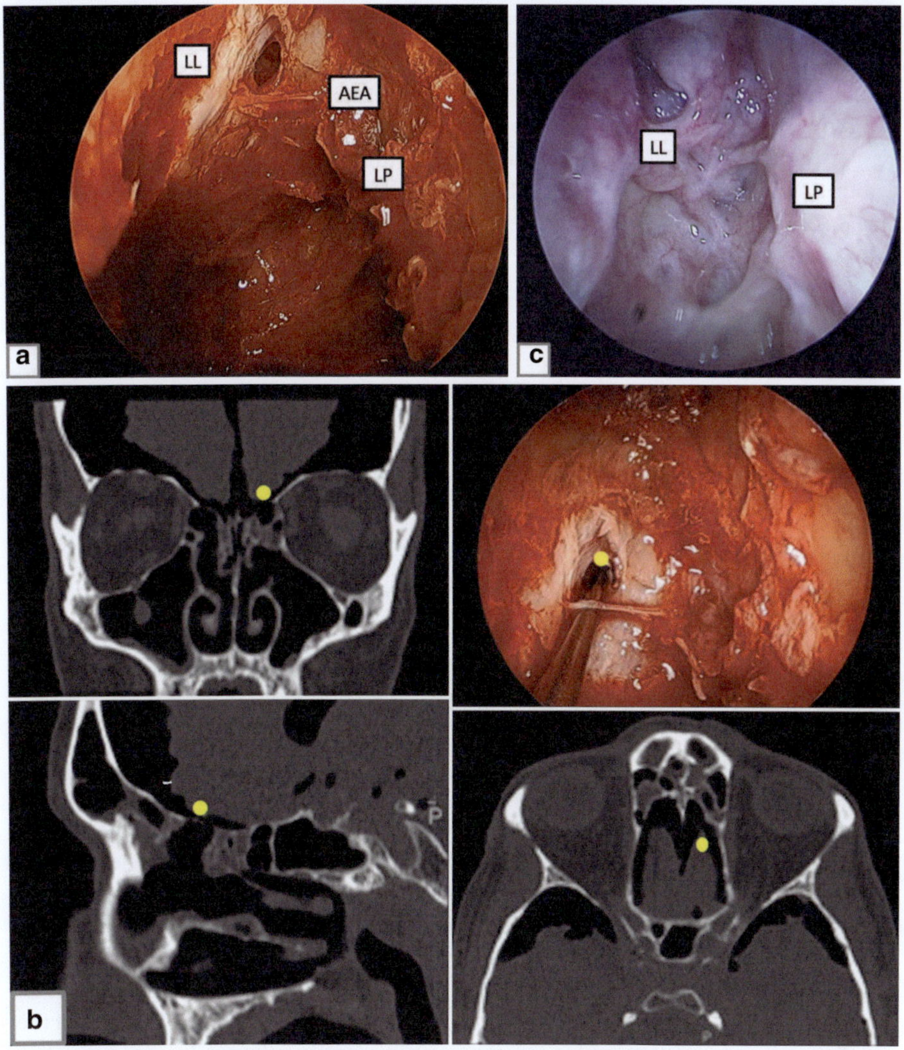

Fig. 11.2 (**a**) Intraoperative endoscopy of skull base defect. Notably, the defect is just anterior and superior to the anterior ethmoid artery (AEA), adjacent to the lateral lamella (LL). The lamina papyracea (LP) is also labeled for orientation. (**b**) Image-guidance navigation (yellow dot) shows probe at the level of the defect along the left lateral lamella in the coronal, axial and sagittal planes of a sinus CT scan. A curved image-guidance probe is shown within the left ethmoid skull base defect in the intraoperative endoscopy view (upper right quadrant). (**c**) Postoperative endoscopy demonstrating excellent repair with re-mucosalization of skull base defect. LL and LP labeled for orientation

Root Cause Analysis

Although iatrogenic CSF leakage can be associated with complicated anatomy or pathology, in this case, the skull base injury was not recognized intraoperatively, suggesting anatomical misunderstanding during the dissection. It is unknown whether stereotactic navigation had been used, but regardless, it is important to note that this adjunctive tool does not replace the surgeon's knowledge of endoscopic sinus anatomy.

Lessons Learned

The present case highlights the need for preparation for this complication, should it occur. Importantly, it also prompts one to consider measures for prevention.

Management of Iatrogenic Cerebrospinal Fluid Leak

The management of an iatrogenic cerebrospinal fluid (CSF) leak depends first on whether the surgeon identifies the leak intraoperatively or, if instead, the leak is noted in a delayed fashion postoperatively. If the surgeon does identify an iatrogenic intraoperative CSF leak during FESS (Fig. 11.3), the first step is to remain calm as this is a readily managed issue with excellent outcomes. One should then communicate the situation with the anesthesiologist, ask for a dose of IV ceftriaxone and level the operating table to reduce the risk of cephalad air entrapment. The nose can then be gently packed and the surgeon can then take the time to re-review the patient's radiographic imaging to better understand the patient's specific skull base anatomy and correlate this with what the surgeon has found intraoperatively, as well as identify any possible preoperative sites of dehiscence of the skull base [1, 2]. After reviewing the imaging, the next step is to identify the skull base defect. At this stage, it may be helpful to widen the exposure to identify relevant landmarks to better understand the intraoperative anatomy. Helpful landmarks during standard FESS include: (i) the superior aspect of the face of the sphenoid sinus where the posterior skull base begins, (ii) the middle turbinate and lamina papyracea that define the medial and lateral corridor of the ethmoid cavity, and (iii) the orbital floor and posterior wall of the maxillary sinus following antrostomy, both of which will always be inferior to the skull base. Next, the surgeon should then examine commonly injured regions of the skull base, including the lateral lamella of the cribriform plate and the fovea ethmoidalis. While hemostasis is important for visualization, it is also important to be cautious when controlling for hemostasis near the skull base defect given the risk of vascular insult to intracranial tissues [2].

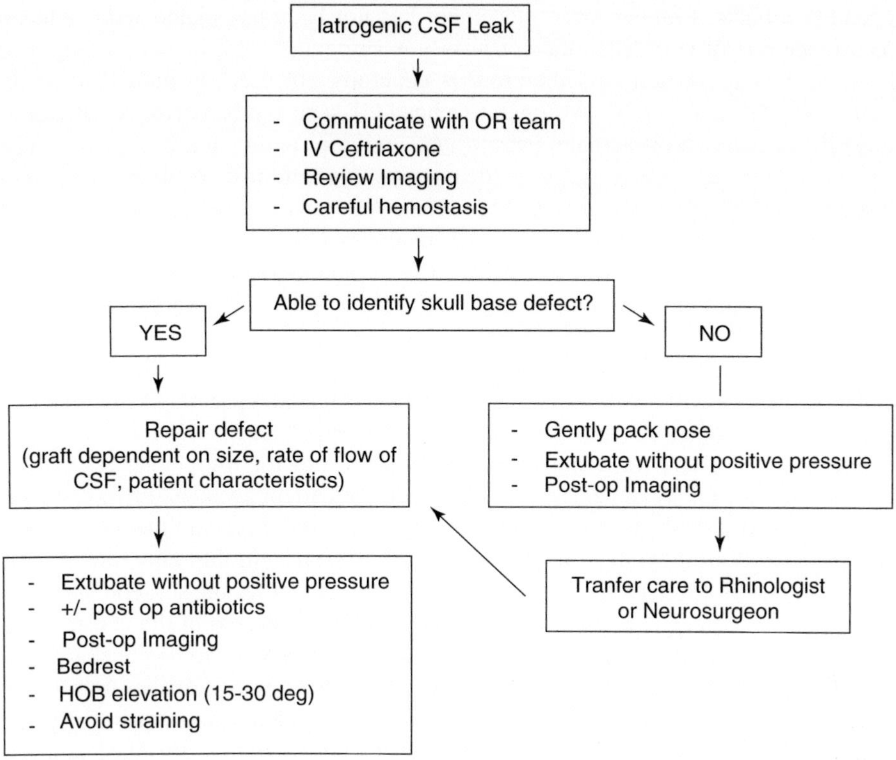

Fig. 11.3 Algorithm for iatrogenic CSF leak noted intraoperatively

Once the skull base defect is identified, the site must be meticulously prepared for coverage via graft or flap tissue. The defect must be fully exposed, with surrounding air cells or intervening structures such as turbinate lamella removed as possible for optimal graft placement. Next, 2–3 mm of the mucosa around the perimeter of the defect should then be removed or stripped to allow the graft full bony contact in a circumferential fashion. The defect is then measured. Various algorithms have been published describing what type of graft is needed for certain sizes of defect. Welch et al. recommends an overlay graft (either free mucosal graft, pedicled mucosal flap or fascia) for defects <2 mm, a composite graft (middle turbinate is often used with a composite of mucosa and bone) for defects between 2–6 mm, and a multilayered closure involving an inlay bone graft (harvested from the septum or mastoid) and onlay mucosal graft (free or pedicled) for defects >6 mm [1]. Following graft positioning over the defect, tissue glue and layers of resorbable packing are typically placed to bolster the graft in situ for several days. Intraoperative antibiotics should be administered, but the need for postoperative antibiotics is controversial [3–6]. After repair, the patient is slowly emerged from general anesthesia to limit coughing or straining. It is also important to communicate with the anesthesia team to avoid the use of positive pressure after extubation, to reduce any risk of pneumocephalus. Lumbar drain placement has not been associated with reduced recurrence rate of CSF leak, and conversely is associated with increased length of inpatient hospitalization, and therefore is generally not used by these authors in iatrogenic CSF leaks [7, 8]. Postoperative head CT scan can be performed to document the absence of intracranial hemorrhage and improving pneumocephalus. The patient should then stay overnight in the hospital to permit in-person disclosure and discussion of the unexpected intraoperative events and corrective measures, and also to monitor neurological status and maintain CSF leak precautions. These include bed rest with head of bed elevated 15–30° and avoiding activities that cause excess straining. Often antiemetics and stool softeners are helpful adjuncts to avoid straining [1, 2].

If the surgeon is unable to identify the defect, it is best to obtain an intraoperative consultation of another otolaryngologist, ideally with a background in rhinology or endoscopic skull base surgery, or a neurosurgeon depending on availability. If the consultant is not able to come to the operating room for immediate repair, the patient's nasal cavity can be gently packed, and the patient awakened from general anesthesia. Communication with anesthesia is necessary to prevent the use of positive pressure during extubation. Postoperative CT scan with thin cuts of the skull base is often helpful to better identify the skull base defect for the surgeon who will perform the repair. The patient will then need to be transferred to the consultant's care for urgent repair in a similar fashion to that described above. If the skull base defect is not readily identifiable on imaging, the surgeon may consider intrathecal injection of low-dose 0.1% fluorescein to identify the defect intraoperatively. Of note, the above is an off-label use of fluorescein and requires informed consent [9, 10].

If the surgeon fails to identify an iatrogenic CSF leak has occurred during the initial operation, the patient is at risk for more serious complications including meningitis and pneumocephalus as well as associated increased medical costs [11]. It is important for otolaryngologists to have a low threshold of suspicion for postoperative complications when patients note red flag symptoms such as copious nasal drainage, unilateral nasal discharge, fever, severe headache, or chills in the postoperative setting. If a postoperative CSF leak is suspected, the next steps include nasal endoscopy to evaluate for CSF leak and direct inspection of the skull base, neurological exam, and CT imaging with fine cuts of the skull base. Collection of nasal discharge fluid for beta-2 transferrin testing can be considered for equivocal cases, but the presence of a steady "leaky faucet" of fluid from the nasal cavity is essentially diagnostic. If a CSF leak is identified or highly suspected, the patient should be admitted to the hospital with plans for urgent repair of the skull base defect. While awaiting repair, patients should be on bed rest with head of bed elevated to 15–30° and be instructed to avoid straining. If a patient presents with fever, leukocytosis, severe headache, or photophobia – ascending infection leading to meningitis should be considered. A lumbar puncture (LP) should be done to culture the CSF prior to starting broad-spectrum antibiotics. Importantly, a lumbar drain, if placed at the time of LP, should not be opened to drain CSF fluid prior to repair for numerous reasons of patient safety and comfort. Only after definitive skull base repair can opening of a lumbar drain be considered. If a patient is found to have pneumocephalus on imaging, patients should be put on 100% supplemental oxygen to facilitate faster reabsorption of pneumocephalus [12], undergo serial neurological exams, and be scheduled for repair urgently. Neurosurgery consultation is also recommended in these patients. As above, close communication with anesthesia is necessary to avoid positive pressure during intubation. Repair should proceed in a similar fashion as described above with similar postoperative care.

How to Prevent Iatrogenic Skull Base Defects

Reported rate of iatrogenic CSF leak during FESS is less than 1%, with most common locations occurring at the lateral lamella, the fovea ethmoidalis, the cribriform plate and the sphenoid sinus [13, 14]. Complication rates will never be completely avoidable, but with comprehensive knowledge of anatomy and an understanding of common pitfalls, the rate of complications can be minimized. Of primary importance is understanding skull base anatomy, which is achieved through a combination of extensive analysis of imaging, cadaver, or simulated dissections prior to surgery near skull base structures, and surgical experience. In a retrospective review of seven patients with skull base injury during FESS, authors found the highest likelihood of skull base penetration was in surgeon inexperience, highlighting the need to be prepared as best as possible prior to embarking on these procedures [15]. Prior to starting a FESS, the surgeon should identify the pertinent landmarks of the individual patient's anatomy including the slope of the skull base, the Keros staging with care to note asymmetry, the location of the anterior ethmoid arteries, the relationship of the frontal recess tract relative to the uncinate, the presence of Onodi cells, possible dehiscence of the optic nerve or internal carotid artery, and air cell developmental complexity of the frontal recess, osteomeatal complex, and the ethmoid cavity. Often surgeons have a routine, methodical way in which they look through a CT scan in order to capture all of this germane information. An image guidance navigation system can be used as a surgical adjunct during FESS, if the surgeon anticipates dissection along the skull base or the patient is undergoing a revision procedure that may result in unusual or altered anatomic relationships.

Recognizing certain pitfalls that may put a patient at greater risk for an iatrogenic CSF leak is also important prior to surgery. Certain anatomical variants may cause a surgeon to be led to the skull base quicker than expected and therefore put patients at risk for an iatrogenic CSF leak. For example, in a retrospective case-controlled study of 18 patients who had iatrogenic CSF leaks during FESS compared to 18 patients who underwent FESS without complication, it was found that in patients who experienced an iatrogenic CSF leak, their skull base had a significantly greater angle in the sagittal plane, a significantly greater slope in the coronal plane, and a significantly lower cribriform plate relative to the ethmoid roof compared to patients who did not experience an iatrogenic CSF leak [16]. Maxillary sinus to ethmoid sinus height has also been noted to be variable – in a review of CT scans from 200

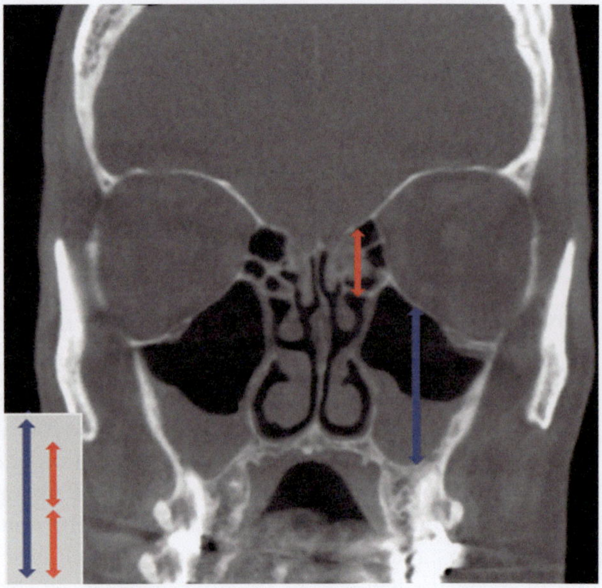

Fig. 11.4 CT scan, coronal view, showing a greater than 2:1 maxillary:ethmoid height ratio. Red arrow demonstrates height of ethmoid cavity. Blue arrow demonstrates height of maxillary sinus. This CT scan image derives from the same patient with the complication described in this chapter. This anatomic ratio was likely not considered and noted by the primary surgeon, contributing to this complication

patients, 58% showed a maxillary: ethmoid height ratio of 1:1, 37% had 2:1, and 5% had >2:1 [17]. This is of particular importance when one is dissecting through the basal lamella of the middle turbinate and entering the posterior ethmoid cavity. In a majority of patients, the ethmoid sinus height is expected to be endoscopically similar to the height of the maxillary sinus. However, in the minority of patients who have limited ethmoid height, a surgeon would be at the skull base sooner than expected, leading to higher risk of violation of the skull base (Fig. 11.4). Significant asymmetry of the skull base, although present in a minority of patients [18], can also lead to higher risk of skull base injury as the surgeon may expect similar height of the skull base on the contralateral side and therefore be unprepared when the skull base is lower than expected. Having an understanding of these less common anatomical variants prompts the surgeon to evaluate these areas on the CT scan prior to beginning FESS to adjust expectations of where the skull base will be in these patients with rare anatomic deviations. With knowledge of the skull base, experience and understanding of common pitfalls, the majority of iatrogenic skull base defects during endoscopic sinus surgery can be avoided.

References

1. Welch KC, Palmer JN. Intraoperative emergencies during endoscopic sinus surgery: CSF leak and hematoma. Otolaryngol Clin N Am. 2008;41(3):581–96.
2. Al-Reefy H, Hopkins C. Up-to-date expert opinion referencing the best evidence available on intraoperative cerebrospinal fluid leak during endoscopic sinus surgery. Clin Otolaryngol. 2013;38(1):48–53.

3. Daudia A, Jones NS. Risk of meningitis with cerebrospinal fluid rhinorrhea. Ann Otol Rhinol. 2007;116:902–5.
4. Brodie HA. Prophylactic antibiotics for posttraumatic cerebrospinal fluid fistulae. A meta-analysis. Arch Otolaryngol Head Neck Surg. 1997;123:749–52.
5. Poletti-Muringaseril SC, Rufibach K, Ruef C, Holzmann D, Soyka MB. Low meningitis-incidence in primary spontaneous compared to secondary cerebrospinal fluid rhinorrhea. Rhinology. 2012;50(1):73–9.
6. Ratilal BO, Costa J, Pappamikail L, Sampaio C. Antibiotic prophylaxis for preventing meningitis in patients with basilar skull fractures. Cochrane Database Syst Rev. 2015;28(4):CD004884.
7. Adams AS, Russel PT, Duncavage JA, Chandra RK, Turner JH. Outcomes of endoscopic repair of cerebrospinal fluid rhinorrhea without lumbar drains. Am J Rhinol Allergy. 2016;30(6):424–9.
8. Caballero N, Bhalla V, Stankiewicz JA, Welch KC. Effect of lumbar drain placement on recurrence of cerebrospinal rhinorrhea after endoscopic repair. Int Forum Allergy Rhinol. 2012;2(3):222–6.
9. Keerl R, Weber RK, Draf W, Wienke A, Schaefer SD. Use of sodium fluorescein solution for detection of cerebrospinal fluid fistulas: an analysis of 420 administrations and reported complications in Europe and the United States. Laryngoscope. 2004;114(2):266–72.
10. Placantonakis DG, Tabaee A, Anand VK, Hiltzik D, Schwartz TH. Safety of low-dose intrathecal fluorescein in endoscopic cranial base surgery. Neurosurgery. 2007;61(3 Suppl):161–5.
11. Li M, Mao S, Tang R, et al. Delayed diagnosis and treatment of cerebrospinal fluid leakage in current practice. J Craniofac Surg. 2019;30(6):1657–61.
12. Gore PA, Maan H, Chang S, Pitt AM, Spetzler RF, Nakaji P. Normobaric oxygen therapy strategies in the treatment of postcraniotomy pneumocephalus. J Neurosurg. 2008;108(5):926–9.
13. Gray ST, Wu AW. Pathophysiology of iatrogenic and traumatic skull base injury. Adv Otorhinolaryngol. 2013;74:12–23.
14. DelGaudio JM, Mathison CC, Hudgins PA. Preoperative disease severity at sites of subsequent skull base defects after endoscopic sinus surgery. Am J Rhinol. 2008;22(3):321–4.
15. Lee JC, Song YJ, Chung YS, Lee BJ, Jang YJ. Height and shape of the skull base as risk factors for skull base penetration during endoscopic sinus surgery. Ann Otol Rhinol Laryngol. 2007;116(3):199–205.
16. Heaton CM, Goldberg AN, Pletcher SD, Glastonbury CM. Sinus anatomy associated with inadvertent cerebrospinal fluid leak during functional endoscopic sinus surgery. Laryngoscope. 2012;122(7):1446–9.
17. Ramakrishnan VR, Suh JD, Kennedy DW. Ethmoid skull-base height: a clinically relevant method of evaluation. Int Forum Allergy Rhinol. 2011;1(5):396–400.
18. Solares CA, Lee WT, Batra PS, Citardi MJ. Lateral lamella of the cribriform plate: a software-enabled computed tomographic analysis and its clinical relevance in skull base surgery. Arch Otolaryngol Head Neck Surg. 2008;134(3):285–9.

Chapter 12
Tension Pneumocephalus

Megan Falls and Jonathan Ting

Clinical Pearls

1. Signs and symptoms of tension pneumocephalus are nonspecific and varied in severity, so the clinician should maintain a high suspicion for tension pneumocephalus in any patient with worsening neurologic symptoms after sinus and skull base surgery.
2. There are several temporizing measures that may be helpful while awaiting definitive closure of the skull base defect including clamping the lumbar drain (if present), bed rest, and avoiding Valsalva-like maneuvers like nose blowing.
3. Definitive management of tension pneumocephalus after sinus or endoscopic skull base surgery requires successful closure of the skull base defect and separation of the intracranial space from the nasal cavity. Intrathecal fluorescein may assist in identifying the site of the leak. The Valsalva maneuver may be helpful intraoperatively to test the integrity of the repair.

Case Presentation

A 72-year-old male had endoscopic sinus surgery (ESS) at an outside hospital for chronic sinusitis with extensive nasal polyposis. This was complicated by an intraoperative cerebrospinal fluid (CSF leak) that was recognized at the time of surgery in addition to a transgression of the lamina papyracea. A left ethmoid cribriform defect was noted and an attempt at intraoperative repair was performed with dural matrix and fibrin sealant in addition to lumbar drain placement by Neurosurgery. Postoperatively, the patient noted horizontal diplopia as well as intermittent but

M. Falls · J. Ting (✉)
Indiana University School of Medicine, Indianapolis, IN, USA
e-mail: megfalls@iu.edu; joting@iu.edu

R. K. Chandra, K. C. Welch (eds.), *Lessons Learned from Rhinologic Procedure Complications*, https://doi.org/10.1007/978-3-030-75323-8_12

persistent unilateral clear drainage. On the evening of postoperative day 2, the patient developed increased drowsiness and altered mental status. Computed tomography (CT) imaging of the brain and sinuses on postoperative day 2 demonstrated increased pneumocephalus (Fig. 12.1). High-flow oxygen delivery was started through a Venturi mask, the lumbar drain was clamped, and the patient transferred to a tertiary care hospital.

Following urgent transfer, the patient was brought to the operating room in the early morning of postoperative day 3 for CSF leak repair. Preoperative CT scan of the sinuses was performed for image guidance (Fig. 12.2). The existing lumbar drain was injected with fluorescein to identify all potential sites of leak, and image guidance was utilized. He was found to have a 1 cm left ethmoid skull base defect. The left middle turbinate was resected for exposure. A graft of DuraGen oversized by approximately 1 cm around the defect was placed in an underlay fashion circumferentially around the defect. A left pedicled septal mucosal flap was then harvested. Next, a septal cartilage graft was harvested and countersunk into the skull base defect. The pedicled septal mucosal flap was then retrieved from its storage location and oriented so its mucosal side faced into the nasal cavity. The flap was then positioned so the entire defect was covered.

The patient's postoperative course after CSF leak repair was uneventful with improved mental status to baseline over several days. Repeat Head CT demonstrated interval decrease of pneumocephalus and the patient was followed for several months with ultimate resolution of his diplopia (Fig. 12.3).

Fig. 12.1 Initial axial CT revealing pneumocephalus

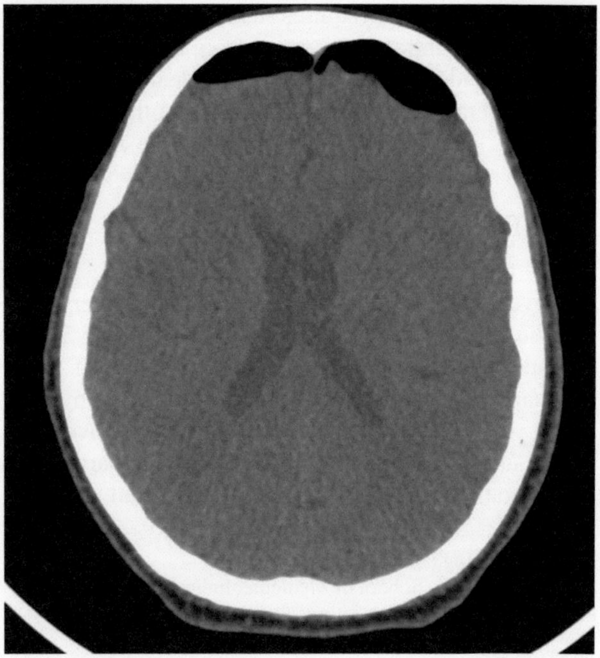

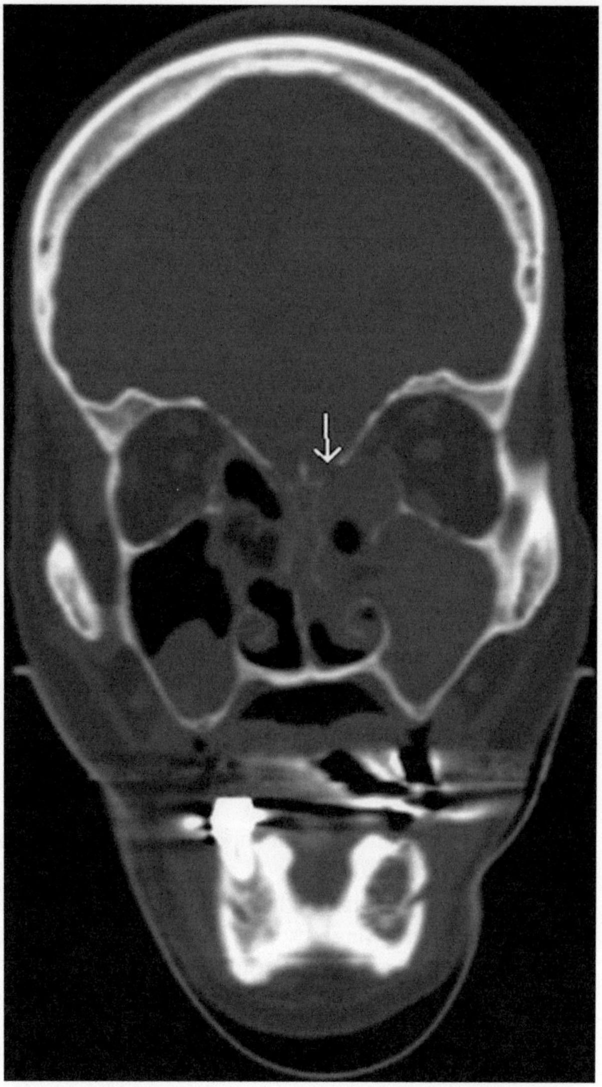

Fig. 12.2 Coronal CT revealing defect in left ethmoid roof

Root Cause Analysis

Tension pneumocephalus is an uncommon complication that may occur following endoscopic sinus or skull base surgery. Postulated mechanisms of tension pneumocephalus may include the "ball-valve" mechanism or the "inverted bottle" mechanism (discussed below). Presence of an open lumbar drain can create a gradient for air influx, particularly in the setting of active nasal airflow.

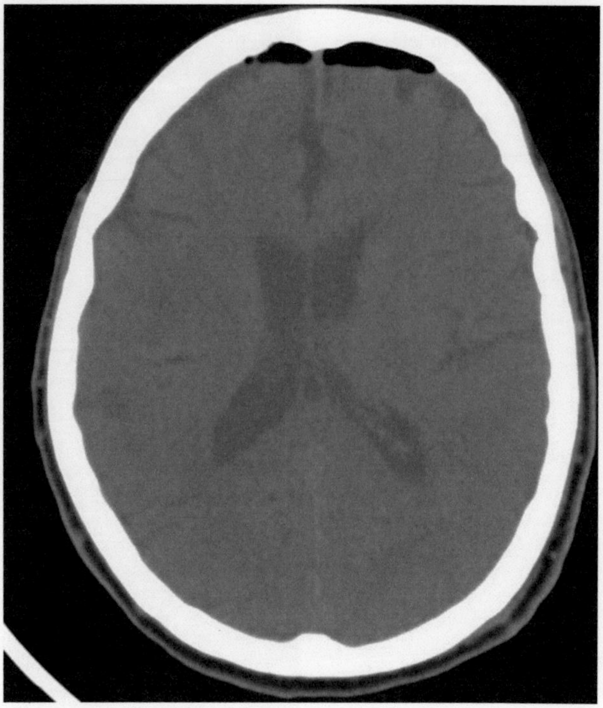

Fig. 12.3 Follow-up axial CT revealing resolving pneumocephalus

Lessons Learned

Tension pneumocephalus is an uncommon complication after endoscopic sinus surgery after unsuccessful repair of a CSF leak. Alternatively, while some degree of pneumocephalus is common in the early postoperative period of expanded endonasal skull base surgery and resolves without treatment, tension pneumocephalus may also occur in this scenario. It is important to maintain a high degree of vigilance as tension pneumocephalus requires prompt intervention with temporizing measures followed by definitive surgical treatment.

Tension pneumocephalus is a result of increased air pressure in the subdural space causing an extra-axial mass effect on the brain [1]. Under normal physiologic conditions, intracranial pressure is higher than atmospheric pressure, so there must be some change in pressures that allows pneumocephalus to develop [2]. There are thought to be two mechanisms of tension pneumocephalus. The first is the "ball-valve" mechanism, where air enters intracranially through a bony defect when the patient has increased nasopharyngeal pressure from actions such as nose blowing, coughing, or sneezing. The outflow of this intracranial air is then obstructed in some fashion, often by the filling of the defect with the surrounding soft tissue [1, 3]. Another mechanism of pneumocephalus is the "inverted bottle" mechanism, which refers to the manner in which lost CSF (whether traumatic or iatrogenic) may draw in air intracranially to replace lost volume [4].

Tension pneumocephalus often develops acutely; the neurological signs and symptoms are presumably related to the compression of brain parenchyma. Symptoms are nonspecific and varied in severity, with headache being the most common of symptoms. Other symptoms include vomiting, visual disturbance, CSF rhinorrhea, altered mental status, and even coma. CT of the brain provides a definitive diagnosis, and nasal endoscopy may be a helpful adjunct to identify the size and location of possible CSF leak. A high index of clinical suspicion is critical in these patients, as tension pneumocephalus has the potential to progress to fatal brainstem herniation if not recognized and treated [2–4].

Recognized causes of tension pneumocephalus are varied but include trauma, prior surgery, sinonasal tumors, and infections. Otolaryngologic procedures that have been reported in the literature to cause pneumocephalus include endoscopic sinus surgery, endoscopic transsphenoidal pituitary surgery, intranasal ethmoidectomy, and less commonly septoplasty [3]. The lateral lamella of the cribiform plate as it attaches to the *fovea ethmoidalis* is the most likely site of iatrogenic injury that results in an intracranial complication such as pneumocephalus [2]. Even a small bony defect of 1 mm has been reported to lead to the accumulation of subdural air and cause tension pneumocephalus [3, 5, 6]. Though exceedingly rare, it is possible that tension pneumocephalus may develop postoperatively in sinus surgery without any obvious skull base defect [3].

The use of nitrous oxide as a neurosurgical anesthetic has been identified as a cause of tension pneumocephalus. Since the blood:gas coefficient of N_2O is almost 34 times more than nitrogen, it diffuses into the subdural space at a rate faster than it is able to be absorbed, which increases postsurgical pneumocephalus [7, 8]. Tension pneumocephalus has been described after hyperbaric oxygen therapy (HBOT) with the theory that air is pulled in through the dural defect due to the negative pressure in the cranium during HBOT. The resulting negative pressure within the cranium results in the expansion of the intracranial air after decompression, once HBOT is complete [8]. CSF leak, skull fractures, and preexisting pneumocephalus should all be considered contraindications to HBOT [9].

Continuous positive airway pressure (CPAP) ventilation may potentially contribute to worsening of pneumocephalus by the mechanism of increasing intrathoracic pressure, decreasing venous return, and thus increasing intracranial pressure in the setting of a preexisting skull base defect or fracture [8]. While practice patterns regarding CPAP usage after nasal surgery vary among otolaryngologists [10], it is likely prudent to avoid positive pressure ventilation in the immediate postoperative period if there is any concern for CSF leakage or pneumocephalus. Traditionally in sinus or skull base surgery, to keep upper airway pressures low and prevent pneumocephalus, nasal packing is placed postoperatively and patients are discouraged from nose blowing, coughing, sneezing, and straining [3]. There is emerging evidence to suggest that early resumption of CPAP following skull base surgery may not have an increased risk of surgical complications, including pneumocephalus [11, 12].

A significant difference in the volume of air on CT between tension and nontension pneumocephalus has not been found [13]. The characteristic, although not pathognomonic, appearance of tension pneumocephalus on CT scan of the brain is the Mount Fuji sign [1, 14]. Bilateral subdural air causes both compression and separation of the frontal lobes. The collapse of the frontal lobes and widening of the space between the tips of the frontal lobes then have the appearance of Mount Fuji [1]. Occasionally, this can be seen as an ipsilateral "mountain" (Fig. 12.4).

The peaking sign is another distinctive CT finding in pneumocephalus where the frontal lobes form a peak in the midline due to bilateral compression and there is no separation between the two lobes (Figs. 12.1 and 12.3). The peak is caused by the entry point of the bridging veins to the superior sagittal sinus. The peaking sign is more common in pneumocephalus than tension pneumocephalus. The Mount Fuji sign tends to suggest that there is a higher subdural pressure than the peaking sign. The air bubble sign may also be present, which consists of multiple air bubbles scattered around the cisterns. This is usually caused by a tear in the arachnoid membrane, and is more common in tension pneumocephalus [13].

Tension pneumocephalus is treatable when recognized in the appropriate time. Temporizing measures are required to stabilize the patient and prevent further decline in neurological condition until the time of definitive repair. If patient condition permits, initial conservative measures should be bed rest, raising the head of the bed, abstaining from Valsalva or other maneuvers that increase intrathoracic pressure, and possible hyperosmolar therapy [5]. Another nonsurgical option is normobaric treatment with 100% FiO_2. However, a patient can only tolerate 100% FiO2 for 24–48 h due to the risk of pulmonary toxicity [5, 15]. Neurosurgical intervention is often, but not always, required as a temporizing measure if conservative measures are inadequate to prevent neurological deterioration [5]. This may encompass craniotomy, drilling burr holes, or ventriculostomy placement [8]. If the patient has

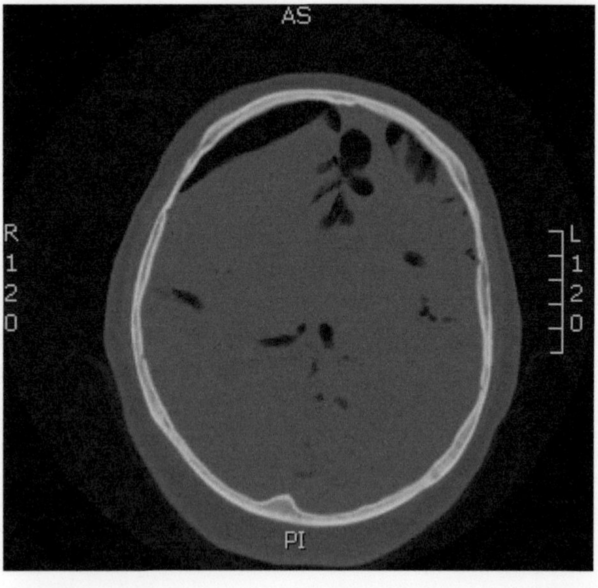

Fig. 12.4 Example of severe pneumocephalus with "mountain" sign on patient's right side

existing burr holes or craniotomy, successful needle decompression with a 22 gauge needle has been described in case reports [4].

Definitive treatment of tension pneumocephalus is repair of the skull base [5, 16]. The use of the Valsalva maneuver intraoperatively is a useful adjunct in repair of CSF leak and skull base defect to adequate repair. The Valsalva maneuver increases intracranial pressure, which promotes spillage of CSF if a non-watertight dural defect still exists [5, 17].

References

1. Michel SJ. The Mount Fuji sign. Radiology. 2004;232(2):449–50.
2. Campanelli J, Odland R. Management of tension pneumocephalus caused by endoscopic sinus surgery. Otolaryngol Head Neck Surg. 1997;116(2):247–50.
3. Whitmore RG, Bonhomme G, Balcer LJ, Palmer JN. Tension pneumocephalus after endoscopic sinus surgery: case report of repair and management in absence of obvious skull base defect. Ear Nose Throat J. 2008;87(2):96–9.
4. Harvey JJ, Harvey SC, Belli A. Tension pneumocephalus: the neurosurgical emergency equivalent of tension pneumothorax. BJR Case Rep. 2016;2(2):20150127.
5. Yin C, Chen BY. Tension pneumocephalus from skull base surgery: a case report and review of the literature. Surg Neurol Int. 2018;9:128.
6. Aksoy F, Dogan R, Ozturan O, Tugrul S, Yildirim YS. Tension pneumocephalus: an extremely small defect leading to an extremely serious problem. Am J Otolaryngol. 2013;34(6):749–52.
7. Artru AA. Nitrous oxide plays a direct role in the development of tension pneumocephalus intraoperatively. Anesthesiology. 1982;57(1):59–61.
8. Pulickal G, Sitoh Y, Ng W. Tension pneumocephalus. Singapore Med J. 2014;55(3):e46–8. https://doi.org/10.11622/smedj.2014041.
9. Lee CH, Chen WC, Wu CI, Hsia TC. Tension pneumocephalus: a rare complication after hyperbaric oxygen therapy. Am J Emerg Med. 2009;27(2):257.e251–3.
10. Cohen JC, Larrabee YC, Weinstein AL, Stewart MG. Use of continuous positive airway pressure after rhinoplasty, septoplasty, and sinus surgery: a survey of current practice patterns. Laryngoscope. 2015;125(11):2612–6.
11. Rieley W, Askari A, Akagami R, Gooderham PA, Swart PA, Flexman AM. Immediate use of continuous positive airway pressure in patients with obstructive sleep apnea following Transsphenoidal pituitary surgery: a case series. J Neurosurg Anesthesiol. 2020;32(1):36–40.
12. White-Dzuro GA, Maynard K, Zuckerman SL, et al. Risk of post-operative pneumocephalus in patients with obstructive sleep apnea undergoing transsphenoidal surgery. J Clin Neurosci. 2016;29:25–8.
13. Ishiwata Y, Fujitsu K, Sekino T, et al. Subdural tension pneumocephalus following surgery for chronic subdural hematoma. J Neurosurg. 1988;68(1):58–61.
14. Biju RD, Wu J, Hussain Z. Tension pneumocephalus after skull base surgery. A case report and review of literature. J Clin Neurosci. 2020;75:218–20. https://doi.org/10.1016/j.jocn.2020.03.041.
15. Hong B, Biertz F, Raab P, et al. Normobaric hyperoxia for treatment of pneumocephalus after posterior fossa surgery in the semisitting position: a prospective randomized controlled trial. PLoS One. 2015;10(5):e0125710.
16. Church CA, Chiu AG, Vaughan WC. Endoscopic repair of large skull base defects after powered sinus surgery. Otolaryngol Head Neck Surg. 2003;129(3):204–9.
17. Haldar R, Khandelwal A, Gupta D, Srivastava S, Rastogi A, Singh PK. Valsalva maneuver: its implications in clinical neurosurgery. Neurol India. 2016;64(6):1276–80.

Chapter 13
A Cerebrospinal Fluid Leak Following Endoscopic Resection of a Frontal Sinus Osteoma

Kevin C. Welch

Clinical Pearls

1. Prevention of cerebrospinal fluid (CSF) leaks during the resection of extradural frontal sinus lesions requires a thorough understanding of anatomy, preoperative imaging, and surgical instrumentation.
2. During the endoscopic resection of frontal sinus osteomas, attention to hemostasis and meticulous surgical techniques should be deployed at all times. When drilling down osteoma lesions, care must be taken to be aware of anatomic limitations that impair smooth and controlled movements of the drill.
3. Managing an iatrogenic dural injury and cerebrospinal fluid leak includes watertight seal, postoperative imaging, and consultations with specialists, such as of Infectious Disease and Neurosurgery.

Case Presentation

A 55-year-old woman presented with a 5–6 month history of focal right frontal pressure that was partially relieved with over-the-counter (OTC) analgesics. She had mild issues with nasal congestion and obstruction; however, she denied discolored nasal discharge or significant problems with her sense of smell. She was evaluated for migraines by a neurologist who ordered an MRI, and this MRI revealed a right frontal sinus osseous lesion that was associated with post-obstructive secretions. She had been treated with antibiotics and steroids by her primary care doctor

K. C. Welch (✉)
Otolaryngology-Head & Neck Surgery, Northwestern University/Northwestern Medicine, Chicago, IL, USA
e-mail: kwelch2@nm.org

R. K. Chandra, K. C. Welch (eds.), *Lessons Learned from Rhinologic Procedure Complications*, https://doi.org/10.1007/978-3-030-75323-8_13

as well as two otolaryngologists. Each otolaryngologist recommended surgery, but recommended a rhinologist perform the procedure.

After taking a thorough history a full workup was performed. Her physical examination was unremarkable, and her nasal endoscopy was unrevealing. A point-of-care CT was obtained during the initial visit, and this revealed an osseous lesion filling the right frontal sinus associated with a post-obstructive fluid (Fig. 13.1). Given the failed response to OTC analgesics and migraine medications, a discussion was held regarding the surgical resection of the osteoma. Both external endoscopic and adjuvant external approaches were discussed with the patient, but the patient desired solely an endoscopic approach. The risks (bleeding, infection, injury to the olfactory region, frontal headaches, CSF leak, and meningitis) of the procedure were discussed at length. Additionally, the possible limitations of endoscopic surgery were discussed – particularly the possibility of being unable to fully resect the tumor.

When the patient was taken to the operating room, she underwent an uneventful anesthetic. Intravenous cefazolin was administered for prophylaxis. Topical decongestion with 1:1000 epinephrine and injections with 1% lidocaine with 1:100,000 epinephrine were used throughout the case to assist with hemostasis. The surgical team consisted of the attending, a rhinology fellow, and a junior resident, who all

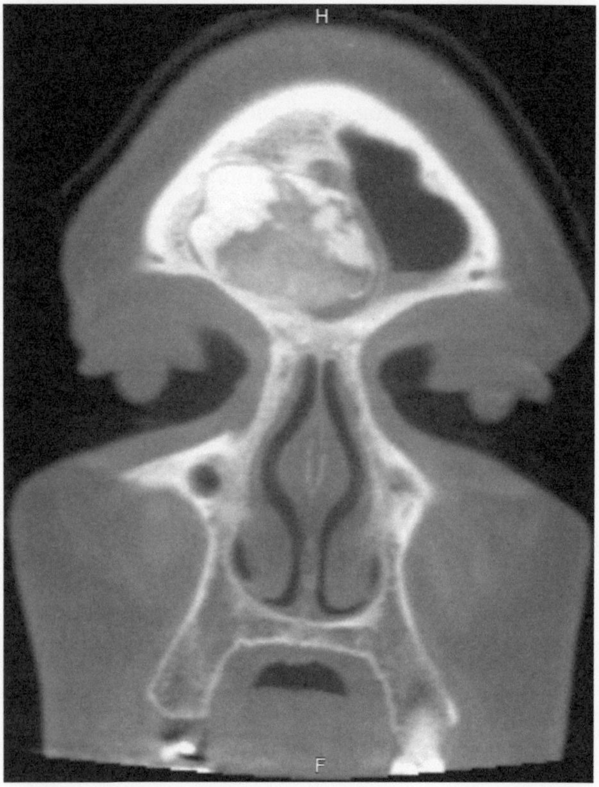

Fig. 13.1 A representative coronal CT image of the patient with a frontal osteoma. A mixed density lesion can be seen occupying the pace of the right frontal sinus with evidence of soft tissue density (likely mucosal thickening) along the medial and inferior aspects of both the right and left frontal sinuses

performed steps of the procedure commensurate with their abilities. Routine bilateral maxillary antrostomies and anterior ethmoidectomies were performed to define the boundaries of the orbit. An anterior-superior septectomy was performed in preparation for a Draf III/modified Lothrop procedure. While using a 70° telescope for visualization, a wide Lothrop procedure was performed, and a combination of drill bits was used to progressively drill down the frontal osteoma. A number of curettes and probes were used to define a plane between the tumor and the anterior and posterior table; however, the tumor was broadly attached to the anterior table, and a plane could not be defined along the posterior table due to angle and instrument limitation. After 4 h of surgery, the apex and lateral aspect of the tumor had been reached. During the drilling, arterial bleeding from the anterior table/anterior portion of the tumor was encountered that was difficult to manage with electrocautery because of the angle. After bleeding was slowed, but not fully controlled, the lateral aspect and superior aspect of the tumor were further resected with a drill. During the drilling, the drill skipped over a portion of the bone, and the lens of the scope became obscured with blood. Drilling was immediately stopped, and after irrigation of the scope, soft tissue consistent with dura and a defect in the posterior table were identified (Fig. 13.2).

At this point, intravenous ceftriaxone was administered, and the surgical site – as well as films – was reexamined. A hemostatic agent was placed into the frontal sinus, and it was lightly packed with saline-moistened pledgets. After all bleeding had subsided and the sinus was thoroughly irrigated, the defect was assessed a second time. There was a 4 mm bony defect and a small dural defect through which there was a slow egress of CSF. An underlay repair was performed using extracellular matrix derived from porcine small intestine submucosa (Biodesign, Cook

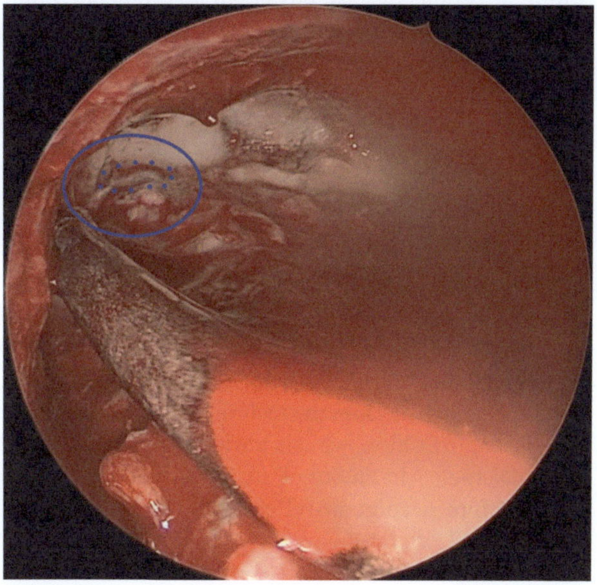

Fig. 13.2 A snapshot of video taken during the procedure. The defect can be seen within the blue oval and more specifically as outlined by the blue dots. In general, the surgical field is remarkable for a partially obstructed view due to bleeding

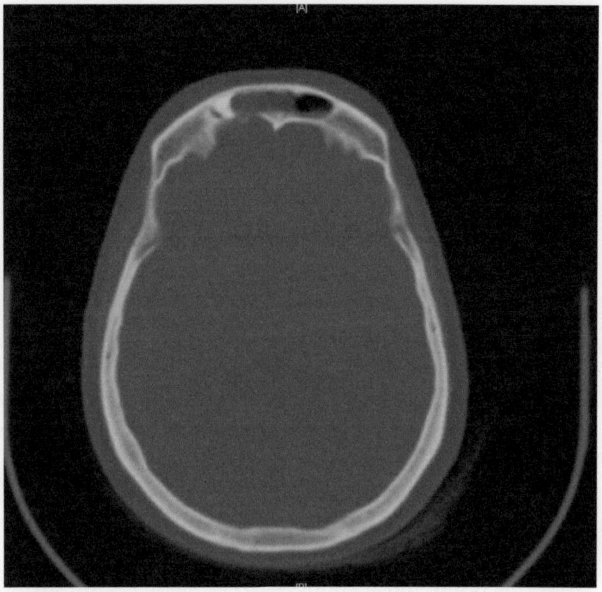

Fig. 13.3 A representative axial CT image of the patient after being recovered and admitted to the hospital. A defect in the posterior wall of the right frontal sinus can be seen with evidence of packing within the frontal sinus. There is no evidence of intracranial blood or air

Medical) and a free bone graft from the posterior septum. An overlay graft consisting of septal mucosa was placed and secured with fibrin sealant. A small pack was placed into the frontal sinus.

The patient was awakened and recovered. A postoperative head CT was obtained and this revealed no pneumocephalus or signs of bleeding (Fig. 13.3). A consulting neurosurgeon recommended no additional investigations or treatments. The consulting infectious disease physician recommended transitioning to oral antibiotics. The patient was discharged on hospital day 2 without further evidence of CSF leak or focal neurological signs and symptoms. The patient's postoperative course with respect to the near-total resection of the tumor and repair of the CSF leak has been unremarkable for the past 2 years. The headaches have resolved.

Root Cause Analysis

Several factors can be considered as being incrementally involved in the cause of this complication. The decision on the approach is the first. The question of whether this surgery should have been done in an open fashion is certainly an important matter of debate. Aside from the technical aspects of performing this surgery in an open or endoscopic fashion, what is the appropriate response to a patient who refuses one particular route? In an era of shared decision-making, how far must the scales be tipped before a surgeon refuses to operate on a patient who has "unrealistic" expectations?

Just prior to the creation of the defect, the surgical team dealt with bleeding that was not completely controlled. The scope tip had blood that obscured the surgeon's view immediately at the time of the injury. To what degree did the bleeding distract the surgical team, or was the skipping of the drill completely unrelated to the distraction of blood? Is there a known relationship between bleeding and additional complications beyond their logical association?

The surgery took 4 h (prior to the repair of the CSF leak) and was the last surgery of the day. To what extent did fatigue play a role in the injury? Factors that led to the length of the surgery included the participation of an otolaryngology resident and rhinology fellow early in his fellowship. At an academic institution, the training of surgical residents is an essential function that attending surgeons perform; however, what is an appropriate amount of involvement? Certainly any resident should be permitted to operate commensurate with his/her abilities and stage, but what is an acceptable prolongation of a surgical case for the benefit of the trainee?

In retrospect, it seems that many of these factors were incrementally involved in the complication; there was not one single event that caused the injury. Rather, the summation of multiple factors resulted in the injury, and each should be examined.

Lessons Learned

The avoidance of complications begins at the onset of the decision for surgery. For every patient who undergoes surgery, a number of initial questions must be answered. Are there any further *appropriate* nonsurgical options? Are there any preexisting medical conditions that may complicate the surgery? What is the appropriate surgical approach/plan for the patient? Does the patient understand the risks, benefits, and alternatives to the surgery? Do the patient and the surgeon agree upon the expectations of surgery? Are there factors (e.g., instruments, staff, surgeon skill set) that limit the ability of the surgeon to safely and successfully complete the surgical task?

In the scenario presented herein, there were no other appropriate nonsurgical options. She had been treated with antibiotics and steroids by three other physicians (two of which were otolaryngologists), and she continued to have symptoms with radiographic evidence of an obstructing lesion with post-obstructive sinus disease. The patient had no preexisting medical conditions that precluded general anesthesia.

The major complication of this case is the CSF leak. It is not a surprise to the reader that a CSF leak would be an expected possible complication associated with the resection of a frontal sinus tumor. Therefore, the repair of the CSF leak itself deserves little attention, as there is a myriad of techniques and methods described that result in adequate repair of dural defects, and multiple studies describe the necessary or recommended postoperative management [1].

The other questions at hand deserve some attention, particularly the decision on the surgical approach. Frontal sinus osteomas have been resected using endoscopic, open and combined approaches for many years, and the choice of which initial approach is appropriate depends on many factors such as tumor size and location. Chiu et al. [2] performed a review of nine patients with frontal sinus osteomas and developed a grading system to help surgeons judge the appropriateness of the endoscopic approach. They concluded that tumors occupying <75% of the frontal recess, having a posterior attachment, and not extending lateral to the lamina papyracea were classified as Grade I tumors. Grade II tumors occupied more than 75% of the frontal recess. Grade III tumors were attached along the anterior table or extended lateral to the lamina papyracea. Grade IV tumors filled the entire sinus. Grade I and II tumors were suitable for endoscopic approaches; however, they concluded that Grade III or IV tumors would need either combined approaches or solely external approaches. In a much larger review, Turri-Zanoni and colleagues [3] reviewed their experience with 60 cases of frontal sinus osteomas. In 31 patients, tumors were resected using a purely endoscopic approach; in 25 cases, a combined open-endoscopic approach was necessary; in four cases, an open approach was used as the sole approach. In patients with extension beyond the lamina papyracea, 31% of tumors were able to be resected using an endoscopic approach alone. These patients had a mix of anterior and posterior attachment sites. The authors ultimately concluded that there were no absolute contraindications to performing a purely endoscopic approach; however, the authors recommended surgeon flexibility to alter the surgical plan during the operation when necessary. In the present case, the patient requested an endoscopic approach with the understanding that there may be an incomplete resection. Adjuvant external approaches were discussed, but the patient declined to consent for those approaches. In an era of shared decision-making, a surgeon may choose to refuse a patient's request or work within the confines of a patient's request. In this author's opinion, if a patient's request does not present a risk to his or her health, it is reasonable to accommodate the patient as long as the limitations and expectations are fully understood.

At the onset of the CSF leak, the surgeons dealt with bleeding from the anterior table that could not be completely controlled but did not completely threaten the surgical field (Boezaart [4] Grade 2). Multiple reports [1, 2, 5, 6] demonstrate the feasibility of endoscopic resection of frontal sinus osteomas, and few document resulting CSF leaks following resection [5–7]. The degree to which the bleeding in this case was associated with the creation of the CSF leak is harder to assess. This author was unable to locate any studies that demonstrated bleeding increases the risk of CSF leak formation in the setting of frontal sinus osteoma resection or in general endoscopic sinus surgery. However, it is logical to conclude that the bleeding was at least a distracting issue that on occasion required disruption of drilling (to suction) and obscured visualization. Therefore, it is recommended that when feasible, minimizing hemorrhage to allow uninterrupted viewing of the operative site be the rule when performing endoscopic sinus surgery.

Another interesting factor to consider and discuss is to what extent this complication was related to the involvement of surgical trainees. Some studies [8, 9] demonstrate that endoscopic sinus surgery is safe in the Academic setting when resident physicians are appropriately supervised; however, in-depth studies as to the techniques of education have not been adequately performed [10]. The part cadaver dissections, simulators, and virtual models play in training may yet prove to reduce even further complications rates. Nevertheless, the successive roles of trainees in this surgical case certainly prolonged the length of the case.

Lastly, does surgeon fatigue increase the risk of complications during endoscopic sinus surgery. All disciplines have investigated the roles sleep deprivation and fatigue play in causing medical errors, and many have opinions. A systematic review by Sturm et al. [11] found some studies that do not show a relationship between fatigue and surgical complications and others that do. Despite widespread investigations that prolonged surgery may result in wound site or hospital-related complications, there is a dearth of data on whether prolonged endoscopic sinus procedures increase the risk of intraoperative complications vis-à-vis surgeon fatigue. Presumably, this would be difficult to study and isolate from general sleep deprivation and fatigue. However, one cannot discount the negative effects prolonged endoscopic sinus surgery and ergonomics has on the surgeon over time [12].

Conclusions

Frontal sinus osteomas can be challenging to manage. While there appear to be few absolute contraindications to an endoscopic approach, the surgeon needs to be flexible about the approach and be able to switch gears during the surgery. When confronted by a patient who strictly wants to avoid any adjuvant external procedures, it is important for the surgeon to understand why and to ensure that the patient has reasonable expectations regarding the potential incompleteness of surgery or any potential increase in complications. Documentation of these discussions is important. Like all cases of iatrogenic CSF leaks, prevention requires understanding of anatomy, control of bleeding, physician attentiveness, and meticulous surgery. Loss of any of those can result in a complication.

References

1. Welch KC, Palmer JN. Intraoperative emergencies during endoscopic sinus surgery: CSF leak and orbital hematoma. Otolaryngol Clin N Am. 2008;41(3):581–96, x. https://doi.org/10.1016/j.otc.2008.01.005.
2. Chiu AG, Schipor I, Cohen NA, Kennedy DW, Palmer JN. Surgical decisions in the management of frontal sinus osteomas. Am J Rhinol. 2005;19(2):191–7. Grading system
3. Turri-Zanoni M, Dallan I, Terranova P, et al. Frontoethmoidal and Intraorbital osteomas: exploring the limits of the endoscopic approach. Arch Otolaryngol Head Neck Surg. 2012;138(5):498–504. https://doi.org/10.1001/archoto.2012.644.
4. Boezaart AP, van der Merwe J, Coetzee A. Comparison of sodium nitroprusside- and esmolol-induced controlled hypotension for functional endoscopic sinus surgery. Can J Anaesth. 1995;42:373–6. https://doi.org/10.1007/BF03015479.
5. Bignami M, Dallan I, Terranova P, Battaglia P, Miceli S, Castelnuovo P. Frontal sinus osteomas: the window of endonasal endoscopic approach. Rhinology. 2007;45(4):315–20.

6. Yiotakis I, Eleftheriadou A, Giotakis E, et al. Resection of giant ethmoid osteoma with orbital and skull base extension followed by duraplasty. World J Surg Onc. 2008;6:110. https://doi.org/10.1186/1477-7819-6-110.
7. Cheng KJ, Wang SQ, Lin L. Giant osteomas of the ethmoid and frontal sinuses: clinical characteristics and review of the literature. Oncol Lett. 2013;5(5):1724–30. https://doi.org/10.3892/ol.2013.1239.
8. Ramadan HH, Allen GC. Complications of endoscopic sinus surgery in a residency training program. Laryngoscope. 1995;105(4 Pt 1):376–9. https://doi.org/10.1288/00005537-199504000-00007.
9. Nguyen QA, Cua DJ, Ng M, Rice DH. Safety of endoscopic sinus surgery in a residency training program. Ear Nose Throat J. 1999;78(12):898–904.
10. Sandhaus H, Chen PG. Intraoperative functional endoscopic sinus surgery training: efficient teaching techniques-a new method. Clin Med Insights Ear Nose Throat. 2018;11:1179550618758647. Published 2018 Mar 5. https://doi.org/10.1177/1179550618758647.
11. Sturm L, Dawson D, Vaughan R, et al. Effects of fatigue on surgeon performance and surgical outcomes: a systematic review. ANZ J Surg. 2011;81(7–8):502–9. https://doi.org/10.1111/j.1445-2197.2010.05642.x.
12. Ramakrishnan VR. Ergonomics in endoscopic sinus surgery. Curr Opin Otolaryngol Head Neck Surg. 2019;27(1):25–8. https://doi.org/10.1097/MOO.0000000000000504.

Chapter 14
Skull Base Injury and Intracranial Complication from Office Sinus Surgery

John M. DelGaudio, Jackson R. Vuncannon, and Emily M. Barrow

Clinical Pearls

1. Procedures utilizing minimally invasive tools still have potential for major complications.
2. Surgical setting, instrumentation, and technique may all be contributing factors in the development of skull base injuries.
3. Failure to recognize the injury and delayed intervention carries a greater risk of dire consequences.

Case Report

A 65-year-old man with a history of sensorineural hearing loss and recurrent otitis externa presented with complaints of otorrhea, nasal congestion, and facial pressure. He was previously treated with two courses of antibiotics for his otitis. In addition, he was administering saline rinses, cetirizine, and fluticasone nasal spray; however, it is unclear if these therapies were targeted to sinonasal complaints as he had no documented history of allergic or rhinologic complaints beyond "mucinous nasal discharge." Computed tomography (CT) imaging of his sinuses demonstrated mucosal thickening in the maxillary sinuses and opacification of the ethmoid and sphenoid sinuses. A recommendation was made for the patient to proceed with office-based endoscopic sinus surgery (ESS). The patient underwent bilateral ethmoidectomy, frontal sinusotomy, sphenoidotomy, and maxillary antrostomy in the office setting under local anesthesia; image guidance was not used. The

J. M. DelGaudio (✉) · J. R. Vuncannon · E. M. Barrow
Department of Otolaryngology, Head and Neck Surgery, Emory University School of Medicine, Atlanta, GA, USA
e-mail: jdelgau@emory.edu; jackson.ross.vuncannon@emory.edu; Emily.barrow@emory.edu

R. K. Chandra, K. C. Welch (eds.), *Lessons Learned from Rhinologic Procedure Complications*, https://doi.org/10.1007/978-3-030-75323-8_14

ethmoidectomy was completed with Blakesly forceps and a microdebrider, while the maxillary, sphenoid, and frontal sinuses were addressed via balloon sinuplasty; placement of the balloon in the frontal sinus was reportedly confirmed by transillumination. The middle turbinates were avulsed with grasping forceps. No complications were noted intraoperatively and the patient was discharged to home from clinic.

On postoperative day 2, the patient reported a fever of 101 °F but was otherwise well. The following afternoon, the patient was found with altered mental status and left hemiplegia and was transported to the hospital. He was admitted to the ICU with concerns for meningitis and stroke as evidenced by elevated lactic acid, tachycardia, fever to 105 °F, and lumbar puncture profile. A CT-head demonstrated pneumocephalus centered over the right frontal lobe and an ipsilateral subdural hygroma measuring 3.6 mm. Intravenous (IV) antibiotic therapy was initiated and Neurosurgery was consulted with recommendations for flat bed rest and serial CT imaging. Magnetic resonance imaging of the brain obtained 24 h later demonstrated persistent pneumocephalus and identified fluid layering in the previously seen subdural collection with adjacent cortical infarcts concerning for empyema (Fig. 14.1). Shortly thereafter, the patient developed seizures and was intubated in the ICU. Neurosurgery performed a craniotomy wherein a large amount of purulence was evacuated from the subdural space and an EVD was placed; the skull base defect was not addressed at this time. A CT-head obtained on the day following this procedure demonstrated resolution of the subdural fluid collection and near complete resolution of pneumocephalus. At no time during the patient's hospitalization was an otolaryngologist involved in his care.

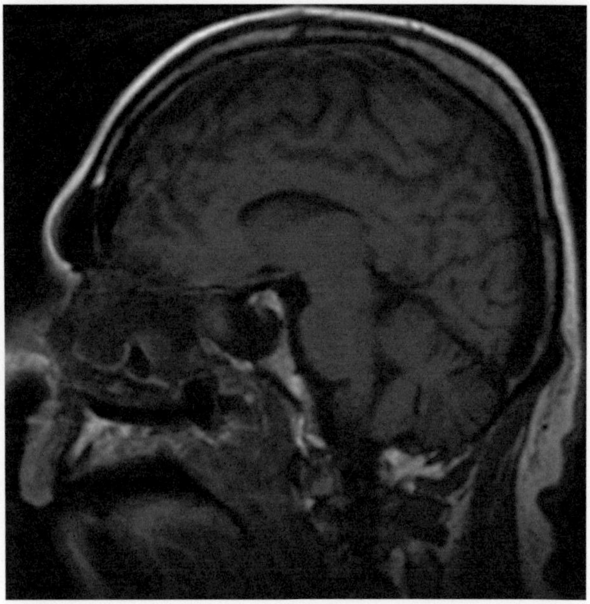

Fig. 14.1 Postoperative MRI, T1 Flair sequence, sagittal section, showing pneumocephalus

The patient continued to improve on IV antibiotics and was ultimately discharged to an inpatient rehabilitation center 15 days following his initial presentation with sepsis; he remained at the rehabilitation center for an additional 35 days and was then discharged to home once functional in activities of daily living. He lives with persistent weakness and paresthesia of the left hand and lower extremity. His skull base defect remains unaddressed.

Root Cause Analysis

In this case, several factors likely contributed to the poor outcome. Although the patient received medical therapy, mostly for otologic complaints, the preoperative CT demonstrates soft tissue density filling the central nasal cavity with peripheral clearing of the sinuses (Fig. 14.2) as well as septal deviation to the right. Further, polyps are clearly seen emanating from the middle turbinates on endoscopy (Fig. 14.3). These findings suggest central compartment atopic disease (CCAD) in an atopic patient [1]. In any event, a thorough history is necessary prior to any surgical intervention. Adequate surgical management of CCAD would include central compartment sculpting, septoplasty (for access and management of the nasal airway), and addressing involved sinuses. While these procedures do not preclude office-based surgery, an operating room would allow a safer and more thorough procedure. Primary balloon sinuplasty is not indicated in the presence of significant polyp disease, except possibly as an adjunct to standard ESS.

In this case, an inappropriate surgical plan was accompanied by poor surgical technique. The ethmoid sinuses were exenterated with grasping instruments with a grasp-and-tear technique. The middle turbinates were avulsed in a similar fashion,

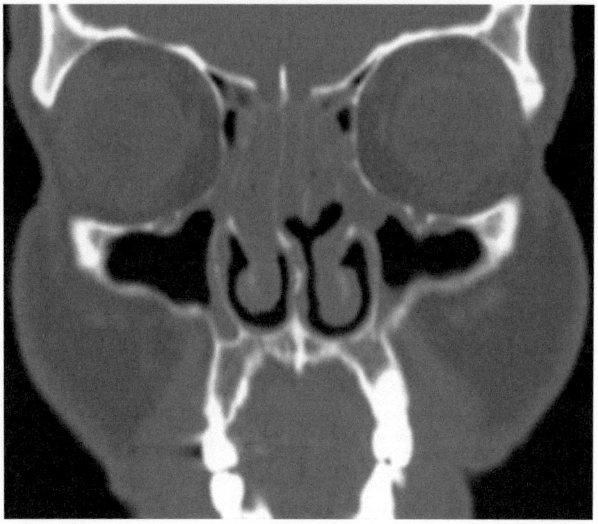

Fig. 14.2 Preoperative CT-sinus, coronal section, shows central compartment soft tissue density with peripheral clearing of the sinuses, consistent with CCAD

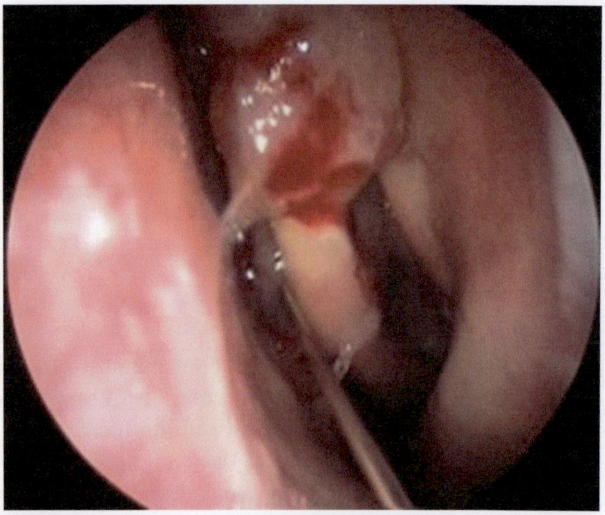

Fig. 14.3 Endoscopic view of left middle turbinate polyp, and polyps medial to middle turbinate. The middle meatus appears free of polyps

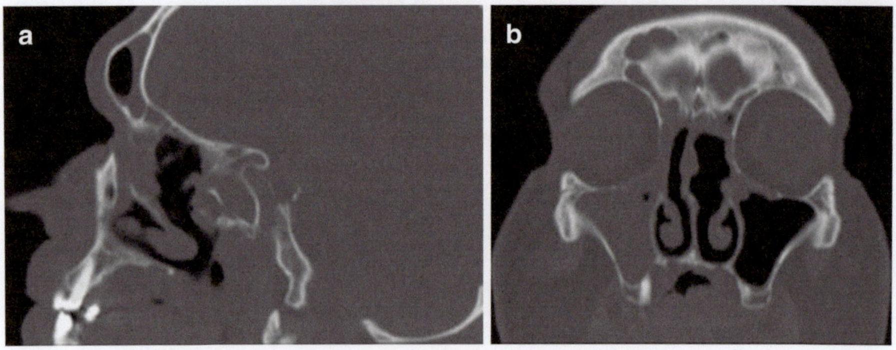

Fig. 14.4 Postoperative CT-sinus, sagittal and coronal section, (**a**) demonstrating remnant agger nasi, and (**b**) showing total middle turbinate resections

either through reckless technique and/or mistaking the turbinate for a polyp. The thin bone of the lateral lamella of the cribriform could easily have been avulsed. There was an incomplete ethmoidectomy, with failure to remove the agger nasi cell (Fig. 14.4), limiting visualization of the skull base and frontal sinus ostium. The nasal septal deviation that was not addressed further reduced access to the right side. Following the traumatic turbinectomy, a combination of powered instrumentation and balloon sinus ostial dilation (BSD) was employed to complete the surgery. The probe for BSD of the frontal sinus was advanced using a 0° endoscope and directed superiorly and medially, instead of a safer lateral angulation. It appears the placement was confirmed by haptic feedback and transillumination rather than precise visualization, as view of the ethmoid roof is potentially limited with the 0° endoscope. It is plausible that the balloon probe was misdirected into a skull base defect produced by the prior MT avulsion or was deflected medially by the remnant agger nasi; alternatively, the balloon could have provided the initial insult to the skull base. However, it is likely that both the MT avulsion and the BSD contributed to the end result. Importantly, no further inspection of the right nasal cavity was undertaken once procedures were begun on the contralateral side, eliminating any opportunity for early identification of a CSF fistula.

The failure to identify this complication in a timely fashion facilitated the progression of ascending meningitis, pneumocephalus, subdural empyema, and stroke with long-term sequelae. Further, the patient continues to live with the skull base defect, which will eventually require additional surgery to repair and will place that patient at risk for further infectious complications.

Lessons Learned

In-Office Management of Sinonasal Disease

Careful attention to patient selection is paramount to successful office-based surgery, with particular consideration given the pathology being managed. Indications for office-based management continue to expand. Authors have thus far reported successful office management of primary and recalcitrant chronic rhinosinusitis, refractory nasal polyposis, sinus recirculation, sinonasal mucoceles, and recurrent inverted papillomas, but the office setting is most commonly employed for sinonasal debridements (99%), polypectomy (77%), and balloon ostial dilations (56%) [2]. Important secondary considerations include factors that could affect visualization such as anatomic abnormalities and the anticipated degree of patient tolerance. Anatomic variations such as deviated nasal septum must be carefully considered not only for their impact on visualization but for their contribution to increased patient discomfort.

Defining criteria for office-based management is an onerous task due to the number of factors that must be weighed. However, ideal patients for office-based procedures possess limited disease in the setting of grossly normal sinonasal anatomy or prior formal ESS. Patient and disease characteristics that discourage an office setting include significant disease burden, pansinuses disease, primary diffuse polyposis, and anatomic abnormalities that may limit visualization. If any of these characteristics are present, careful thought should be given to an operating room setting for more complete management.

In the absence of guidelines, responsibility lies with the surgeon to critically evaluate every patient considered for office-based surgery with regard to one's objective findings and skill set. It is important to recognize this, as a simple and straightforward procedure in the operating room may become substantially more difficult in the office setting. It must also be emphasized that goals of surgery, when done in an office setting, should not deviate from those if done in the operating room merely in an effort to minimize the risks of complications. The surgeon must also have the humility to decide if these goals cannot be accomplished in an office setting, which may require premature termination of the procedure and rescheduling in the operating room.

Balloon Sinus Ostial Dilation

In 2005, the FDA approved balloon sinus ostial dilation (BSD) as a diagnostic and therapeutic approach to the paranasal sinuses. BSD can be used as a "stand-alone" device or in a "hybrid" fashion in conjunction with more traditional sinus instrumentation. BSD has been marketed to shorten recovery time, preserve the nasal mucosa and minimize postoperative care, with additional benefit of ability to be performed in the office setting under local anesthesia [3, 4]. These factors, combined with reimbursement rates for balloon procedures approximately five to ten times greater than for ESS, have led to concerns of overutilization and possibly inappropriate use of these devices [4]. Studies demonstrating the significantly increased rate of BSD since the introduction of CPT codes for these procedures in 2011, without a proportional increase in non-balloon procedures, highlight these concerns [4].

With national practice patterns in balloon sinuplasty varying widely, and aforementioned concerns regarding inappropriate use, the American Academy of Otolaryngology – Head and Neck Surgery published a clinical consensus statement on its usage [5]. While a complete review of the clinical consensus statement guidelines is outside the scope of this review, several guidelines are salient to this case. The overall consensus states that balloon dilation can be appropriate as an adjunctive procedure to ESS in patients with chronic rhinosinusitis (CRS) without nasal polyposis, with near consensus for patients with limited sinus disease who met criteria for surgery prior to considering more extensive sinus surgery. There was no consensus on utilization of BSD either as a sole procedure or as an adjunctive procedure in patients with nasal polyposis (CRSwNP). Furthermore, there was near consensus that balloon dilation of the peripheral sinuses is not effective for managing ethmoid sinusitis. While the ethmoid sinuses are the most common site of disease in CRS, balloon catheters are only available for the frontal, maxillary, and sphenoid sinuses. In light of device constraints and consensus statements, it is generally inadvisable to perform BSD either as the sole procedure or as an adjunct procedure to ESS in patients with CRSwNP and/or ethmoid disease [5].

While BSD is considered safe as a stand-alone or hybrid procedure, complication rates have varied with time [6]. Early studies reported minimal to no adverse events associated with balloon dilation, portraying decreased risks associated with BSD in comparison to traditional ESS [7]. However, many of these studies had strict exclusion criteria excluding patients with extensive sinonasal disease, polyps, prior sinonasal surgery, severe osteoneogenesis, sinonasal malignancy, history of facial trauma, and cystic fibrosis. Subsequent studies of BSD in real-world environments have reported higher rates of complications [8, 9]. A balloon sinus dilator, if introduced incorrectly, can create submucosal false passages or fracture the bone of the ethmoid roof or orbital wall. In fact, complications of BSD may still be underreported as it is often difficult to determine the exact source of injury in hybrid procedures (e.g., whether due to use of the balloon vs. powered dissectors) due to limited dissection of the surrounding sinus ostium [6]. A contemporary analysis of 16,040 patients undergoing sinus surgery, in which 2851 underwent BSD alone, 11,955 underwent conventional FESS, and 1234 underwent a hybrid procedure, found skull base/central nervous system complications occurred in 0.35%; there was no difference in complication rates between patients undergoing FESS or BSD [8].

Timely Identification and Repair of Skull Base Injury

Injury to the anterior skull base with cerebrospinal fluid (CSF) fistula is thus a rare but significant complication of both traditional ESS and BSD and has been reported as the most common cause for litigation following ESS [10]. More importantly, this complication portends a risk for potentially devastating neurologic sequelae. Injury to intracranial structures, intracranial hemorrhage, pneumocephalus, and ascending meningitis have all been reported following skull base violation during ESS [11]. Even in the absence of acute intracranial injury, the risk of meningitis persists. Daudia et al. followed 111 patients with CSF rhinorrhea over a 12-year period and found the overall risk of meningitis was 22% in patients with iatrogenic CSF leak, and this risk was greatest in the first year following the insult [12].

The risk of meningitis can be mitigated through early identification and management of skull base injuries. A large meta-analysis found that endoscopic repair of CSF fistula was associated with a decrease in the annual risk of meningitis from 10% to 0.3% [13]. Additionally, prior case reports have suggested that the morbidity associated with skull base injury during ESS may be related to delayed diagnosis [14]. Kubik et al. specifically investigated the incidence of neurologic sequelae with respect to the timeliness of CSF leak repair in 17 patients; in only three cases was the skull base injury identified intraoperatively. These authors found no cases of meningitis occurred when the leak was identified within 72 hours but meningitis developed in 72.7% (8/11) of cases diagnosed after that time [15]. It is therefore critical to recognize and repair these defects promptly to decrease the risk of complications and neurological sequelae.

Summary

In the case under discussion, a series of errors in surgical planning and technique led to significant patient harm. Nonoptimal surgical setting, inappropriate instrumentation, and failure to differentiate among CRS endotypes or recognize anatomic abnormalities set the stage for a difficult procedure. Visualization was further impacted by imprecise tissue manipulation with resultant bleeding obscuring sinus ostia and, ultimately, the skull base injury. While office-based surgery and BSD have advantages for select patients, it is important to recognize their limitations. A straightforward procedure in the operating room may become substantially more difficult in the office setting. Finally, meticulous surgical technique is necessary in every procedure to protect those in our care.

References

1. DelGaudio JM, Loftus PA, Hamizan AW, Harvey RJ, Wise SK. Central compartment atopic disease. Am J Rhinol Allergy. 2017;31(4):228–34.
2. Lee JT, DelGaudio J, Orlandi RR. Practice patterns in office-based rhinology: survey of the American Rhinologic Society. Am J Rhinol Allergy. 2019;33(1):26–35.
3. Stewart AE, Vaughan WC. Balloon sinuplasty versus surgical management of chronic rhinosinusitis. Curr Allergy Asthma Rep. 2010;10(3):181–7.
4. Calixto NE, Gregg-Jaymes T, Liang J, Jiang N. Sinus procedures in the Medicare population from 2000 to 2014: a recent balloon sinuplasty explosion. Laryngoscope. 2017;127(9):1976–82.
5. Piccirillo JF, Payne SC, Rosenfeld RM, Baroody FM, Batra PS, DelGaudio JM, et al. Clinical consensus statement: balloon dilation of the sinuses. Otolaryngol Head Neck Surg. 2018;158(2):203–14.
6. Alam ES, Hadley JA, Justice JM, Casiano RR. Significant orbital and intracranial complications from balloon sinus dilation as a stand-alone and powered dissector-assisted procedure. Laryngoscope. 2018;128(11):2455–9.
7. Bolger WE, Brown CL, Church CA, Goldberg AN, Karanfilov B, Kuhn FA, et al. Safety and outcomes of balloon catheter sinusotomy: a multicenter 24-week analysis in 115 patients. Otolaryngol Head Neck Surg. 2007;137(1):10–20.
8. Chaaban MR, Rana N, Baillargeon J, Baillargeon G, Resto V, Kuo YF. Outcomes and complications of balloon and conventional functional endoscopic sinus surgery. Am J Rhinol Allergy. 2018;32(5):388–96.
9. Hur K, Ge M, Kim J, Ference EH. Adverse events associated with balloon sinuplasty: a MAUDE database analysis. Otolaryngol Head Neck Surg. 2020;162(1):137–41.
10. Lynn-Macrae AG, Lynn-Macrae RA, Emani J, Kern RC, Conley DB. Medicolegal analysis of injury during endoscopic sinus surgery. Laryngoscope. 2004;114(8):1492–5.
11. Stankiewicz JA, Lal D, Connor M, Welch K. Complications in endoscopic sinus surgery for chronic rhinosinusitis: a 25-year experience. Laryngoscope. 2011;121(12):2684–701.
12. Daudia A, Biswas D, Jones NS. Risk of meningitis with cerebrospinal fluid rhinorrhea. Ann Otol Rhinol Laryngol. 2007;116(12):902–5.
13. Hegazy HM, Carrau RL, Snyderman CH, Kassam A, Zweig J. Transnasal endoscopic repair of cerebrospinal fluid rhinorrhea: a meta-analysis. Laryngoscope. 2000;110(7):1166–72.
14. Hassab MH, Eweiss AZ, Ibrahim AA. Missed skull base injury during sinonasal surgery: a dangerous scenario still existing. Ear Nose Throat J. 2015;94(8):E37–42.
15. Kubik M, Lee S, Snyderman C, Wang E. Neurologic sequelae associated with delayed identification of iatrogenic skull base injury during endoscopic sinus surgery (ESS). Rhinology. 2017;55(1):53–8.

Chapter 15
Penetrating Skull Base Injury and Postoperative Infection

Nikita Chapurin and Rakesh K. Chandra

Clinical Pearls

1. Penetrating skull base injuries require a prompt workup in collaboration with Neurosurgery and removal of the impaled object in a controlled setting, ideally under direct visualization.
2. Intracranial organic foreign objects pose a significant risk of meningitis and abscess formation. These infections are unlikely to clear with antibiotics alone and require meticulous removal of debris.
3. CSF leaks are expected with these injuries, and comprehensive skull base reconstruction should be performed using vascularized native tissue when possible.

Case Presentation

A 65-year-old male with past medical history of atrial fibrillation on Warfarin sustained a fall resulting in impalement of a wood stick through the oral cavity and into the anterior cranial fossa. The object entered the gingivolabial sulcus and passed through maxillary and ethmoids sinuses penetrating the anterior skull base, extending intracranially to corpus callosum (Figs. 15.1 and 15.2). The patient was neurologically intact upon presentation, with normal vision, and did not have a frank CSF leak. Urgent CT angiogram was obtained and showed displacement of anterior cerebral arteries without visible

N. Chapurin
Department of Otolaryngology – Head and Neck Surgery, Vanderbilt University Medical Center, Nashville, TN, USA

R. K. Chandra (✉)
Otolaryngology-Head & Neck Surgery, Vanderbilt University Medical Center, Nashville, TN, USA
e-mail: rakesh.chandra@vumc.edu

R. K. Chandra, K. C. Welch (eds.), *Lessons Learned from Rhinologic Procedure Complications*, https://doi.org/10.1007/978-3-030-75323-8_15

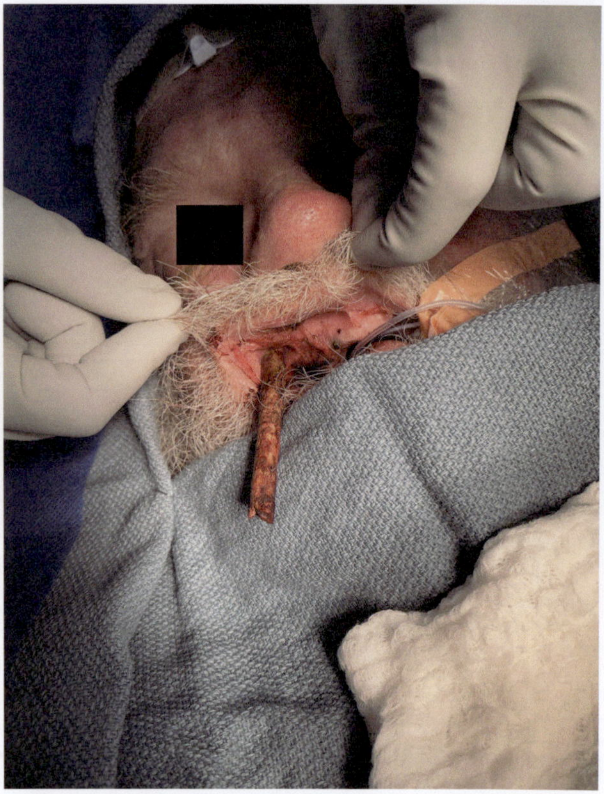

Fig. 15.1 Intraoperative image demonstrating the impaled foreign body entering the oral cavity

vessel injury (Fig. 15.3). After discussion with Neurosurgery, his anticoagulation was reversed, and he was emergently taken to the operating room for controlled removal of foreign body and skull base repair under endoscopic guidance, and possible craniotomy.

To obtain adequate exposure for controlled removal, total sphenoethmoidectomy was performed to expose the object and skeletonize the skull base around it (Fig. 15.4), after which it was carefully withdrawn. It was mostly removed as a single piece, but there were multiple bone fragments and splinters through the impalement site that also extended intracranially that were meticulously removed under endoscopic visualization. There was an expected CSF leak but no significant bleeding. The skull base defect was repaired with an abdominal fat graft placed above the level of the cranial base to close the dead space, and an overlying pedicled mucoperiosteal septal flap, based on the posterior septal branches of the sphenopalatine neurovascular bundle.

Infectious Disease was consulted on postoperative day 1, and patient was empirically started on IV vancomycin and cefepime. Despite no growth of CSF cultures, the decision was made to complete a 10-day course of broad-spectrum antibiotics. On post-op day 10, patient was found to have an altered mental status and was showing a clinical picture of meningitis. Brain MRI (Fig. 15.5) demonstrated a developing abscess in the inferior right frontal lobe, which extended into the corpus

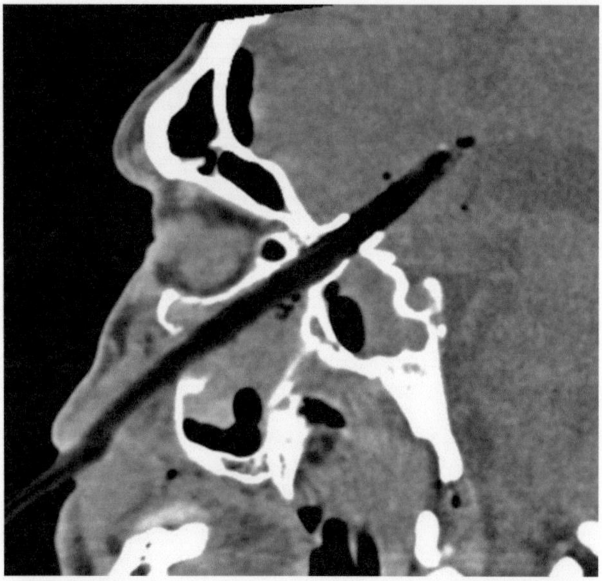

Fig. 15.2 Sagittal view of maxillofacial CT demonstrating the object passing through maxillary and ethmoid sinuses, anterior skull base, and extending intracranially to corpus callosum

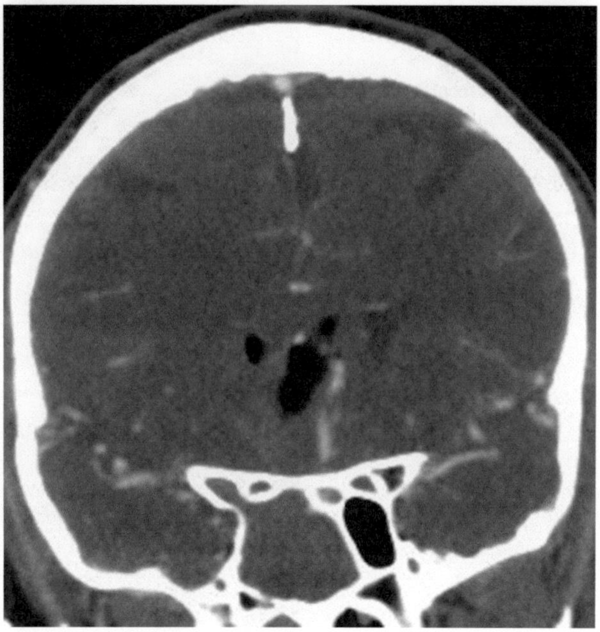

Fig. 15.3 Coronal view of CT head angiogram demonstrating anterior cerebral artery A2 and A3 vessels being displaced to the left by the foreign body, without visible injury

callosum rostrum and genu, along the path of the prior foreign body, and measured 2.7 × 3.8 cm. A ventriculostomy catheter was placed by Neurosurgery, and meropenem was added for enhanced anaerobic coverage. The patient then quickly recovered. His external ventriculostomy device (EVD) was removed, and he was

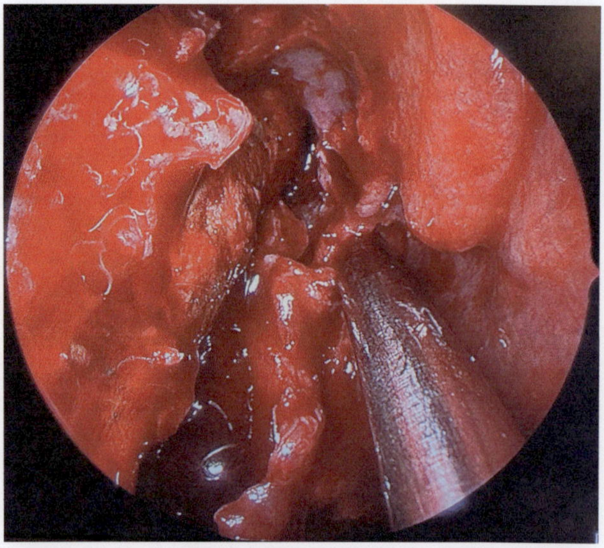

Fig. 15.4 Endoscopic view of the skull base after total sphenoethmoidectomy was performed, demonstrating the object entering the anterior cranial fossa

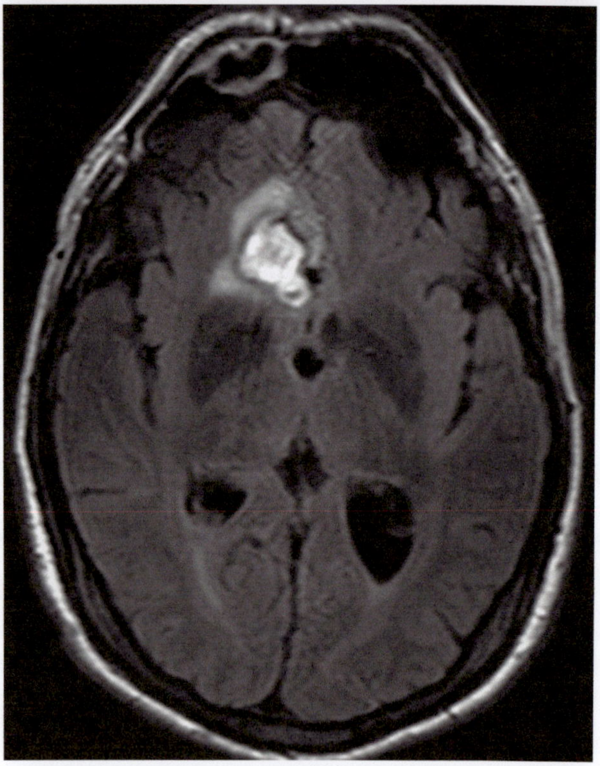

Fig. 15.5 MRI brain with constrast T2 weighted image demonstrating a 3.8 cm abscess in the inferior right frontal lobe that extends into the corpus callosum along the path of the prior foreign body

discharged 3 weeks after his injury. Antibiotics were continued for a 4-week course, and the patient had a full recovery with no recurrence of the CSF leak, signs of central nervous system infection, vision compromise, or neurologic deficits.

Root Cause Analysis

This case demonstrates the complexity of caring for a patient with a penetrating skull base injury. Root causes include: (1) impalement of skull base by unsterile organic foreign body in multiple fragments, which passed through oral cavity and sinuses to reach intracranial space; (2) presence of extensive skull base defect and CSF leak; and (3) inability of antibiotics alone to prevent meningitis.

Complicating factors in management of this patient included (1) anticipation of possible devastating vascular injury; (2) importance of close collaboration with Neurosurgery, Intensive Care Unit (ICU), and Infectious Disease colleagues; (3) need for comprehensive skull base repair with both abdominal fat and vascularized mucoperiosteal septal flap.

Lessons Learned

Endoscopic repair of skull base defects and CSF leaks has been demonstrated to have superior efficacy and decreased morbidity in comparison to open craniotomy approaches [1]. Hence, patients with traumatic skull base injuries are frequently managed by rhinologists, but ultimately require an interdisciplinary approach and close collaboration with Neurosurgery, Neuro-Intensive Care Unit, and Infectious Disease specialists. The team should be prepared to act quickly. It is important to obtain a thorough neurological examination, visual acuity exam, and to evaluate for a potentially devastating vascular injury. Time permitting, it is helpful to also obtain a preoperative CT angiogram or intraoperative angiogram to assess potential injury to cerebral vasculature and their proximity to the foreign object. The patient should be taken to the operating room and foreign object be carefully withdrawn under direct visualization in a controlled environment. Neurosurgery should be also involved in the case and be prepared to perform a craniotomy or endovascular procedure in case of life-threatening complications, such as arterial bleeding and herniation. In this case there was no significant vascular injury and the defect could be repaired endoscopically, so craniotomy could be avoided.

Intracranial infections in the setting of organic foreign bodies are known to be refractory to intravenous antibiotic therapy alone. Literature on traumatic injuries resulting from intracranial wooden foreign bodies has been mostly based on studies of children who fell while carrying sharp objects such as pencils or chopsticks. In the largest series of 42 patients that spanned both the pre- and post-antibiotic era, 48% of the patients developed an intracranial abscess [2]. Among patients in the post-antibiotic era, infection complicated 64% of the cases and there was 25% mortality. There are multiple reasons why wood is particularly prone to infection, including its porous quality and predisposition to fragmentation. The most common organisms found in cultures from these patients were *Staphylococcus aureus*, β-hemolytic streptococci, and *Streptococcus pneumoniae* [3]. Development of biofilms in foreign objects also makes clearing of infections with antibiotics challenging [4]. Therefore, development of meningitis and intracranial abscess, as seen in our patient, should be anticipated and managed promptly. Care must be made to meticulously remove all the impaled foreign bodies to the maximum degree possible without causing further intracranial damage. Patients should be started on broad-spectrum antibiotics under Infectious Disease guidance, and despite potentially negative CSF cultures, as seen in this patient. Clinicians should also anticipate a potentially prolonged course (4 weeks in this patient) to prevent recurrence. Neurosurgical intervention, in form of ventriculostomy or craniotomy, may also be necessary during the course of management.

Management of an expected CSF leak requires preparation for multiple reconstructive options, and consideration of external ventricular drain placement for CSF diversion. Abdominal fat was used in this patient and was favored given the ability to provide a biologic seal with native tissue. The authors suggest avoiding alloplastic materials in these situations, where the complicating factors already relate to organic foreign body. In addition, utilization of vascularized tissue for coverage of the obliterated dead space is likely increases likelihood of successful repair, and prevents recurrent CSF leakage or further contamination of intracranial space [5]. External ventricular drain was also placed by Neurosurgery for CSF diversion and management of potential infection.

Conclusion

Penetrating skull base injuries of this nature require prompt management for potentially devastating injuries, an interdisciplinary approach, and removal under direct visualization in a controlled setting. Organic foreign body impalement carries significant risk of meningitis and abscess formation. Therefore, meticulous removal of all debris and comprehensive skull base reconstruction are critical in mitigating complications.

References

1. Hegazy HM, Carrau RL, Snyderman CH, Kassam A, Zweig J. Transnasal endoscopic repair of cerebrospinal fluid rhinorrhea: a meta-analysis. Laryngoscope. 2000;110(7):1166–72.
2. Miller CF, Brodkey JS, Colombi BJ. The danger of intracranial wood. Surg Neurol. 1977;7(2):95–103.

3. Wieland AM, Curry WT, Durand ML, Holbrook EH. Management of a long-standing organic intracranial foreign body. Skull Base. 2010;20(6):487–90. https://doi.org/10.1055/s-0030-1261264.
4. Sharma D, Misba L, Khan AU. Antibiotics versus biofilm: an emerging battleground in microbial communities. Antimicrob Resist Infect Control. 2019;8:76.
5. Oakley GM, Orlandi RR, Woodworth BA, Batra PS, Alt JA. Management of cerebrospinal fluid rhinorrhea: an evidence-based review with recommendations. Int Forum Allergy Rhinol. 2016;6(1):17–2.

Part III
Surgical Bleeding

Chapter 16
Concentrated Epinephrine Use in the Operating Room

Seth J. Davis, Kyle S. Kimura, William G. Morrel, Raj D. Dedhia, and Scott J. Stephan

Clinical Pearls

1. Methods to avoid accidental injection of concentrated epinephrine:
   - Pre-label all syringes used to draw up any injectable medication.
   - Ask for injectable medications by name, and verify dosages whenever they are transferred between individuals.
   - Use pre-dosed syringes or single dose vials of appropriate concentrations of epinephrine in situations where appropriate.
   - Dispense 1:1000 (1 mg/mL) epinephrine for topical use into a separate container with fluorescein to differentiate from injectable epinephrine-containing solutions.

S. J. Davis (✉) · K. S. Kimura · W. G. Morrel
Department of Otolaryngology – Head & Neck Surgery, Vanderbilt University Medical Center, Nashville, TN, USA
e-mail: seth.davis@vumc.org; kyle.s.kimura@vumc.org; will.morrel@vumc.org

R. D. Dedhia
Department of Otolaryngology, University of Tennessee Health Science Center, Memphis, TN, USA

Division of Facial Plastic and Reconstructive Surgery, University of Tennessee Health Science Center, Memphis, TN, USA
e-mail: raj.dedhia@uthsc.edu

S. J. Stephan
Department of Otolaryngology – Head & Neck Surgery, Vanderbilt University Medical Center, Nashville, TN, USA

Division of Facial Plastic and Reconstructive Surgery, Vanderbilt University Medical Center, Nashville, TN, USA
e-mail: stephan@vumc.org

R. K. Chandra, K. C. Welch (eds.), *Lessons Learned from Rhinologic Procedure Complications*, https://doi.org/10.1007/978-3-030-75323-8_16

2. Recognition and treatment of epinephrine toxicity:
   - Early clinical signs include headache, dizziness, nausea, palpitations, tremor, and generalized weakness.
   - In the OR, hypertension, tachycardia, arrhythmias, and signs of local tissue ischemia should raise suspicion.
   - Initial treatment should focus on control of blood pressure to avoid intracranial hemorrhage and cardiac arrhythmias or arrest.
   - Avoid pure beta blockade that weakens cardiac contractility and can precipitate heart failure.

Case Presentation

A 16-year-old male with history of nasal obstruction secondary to acquired traumatic deformity was scheduled for outpatient external approach septorhinoplasty and inferior turbinate reduction. Preoperative exam was unremarkable, and the case was cleared to proceed by both the surgical and anesthesia teams. Following routine induction of general anesthesia and endotracheal intubation, the surgeon was handed an unlabeled syringe for local anesthetic infiltration of the external nose, turbinates, and septum. This syringe contained only 3 mL of clear fluid which the surgeon noted at the time, commenting that the team would eventually require more local anesthetic. After preoperative timeout was performed, the anesthesia team was notified that "lidocaine with epinephrine" was being injected locally. Following a brief delay, the scrub tech exclaimed that they had accidentally given the surgeon the incorrect syringe – instead of 1% lidocaine with 1:100,000 epinephrine, the surgeon had been given a syringe containing 1:1000 epinephrine. The injection was immediately discontinued after an estimated 0.8 mL had been injected into the right inferior turbinate. The anesthesia team was quickly notified of the situation and the head of the turbinate was incised with a 15-blade in an attempt to express any residual epinephrine before it was absorbed systemically.

Shortly following injection, the patient experienced a rapid spike in blood pressure from 91/58 to 202/125, accompanied by mild ST depression and T-wave inversion on EKG tracing. This was immediately treated with Propofol bolus and increased sevoflurane concentration by the anesthesia team. A blood gas and troponin I were obtained shortly thereafter. Approximately 2 min following initiation of treatment, blood pressure had decreased to 158/79 and cardiac rhythm had normalized. At approximately 7 min following initial injection, blood pressure had returned to near-baseline at 106/42 (Fig. 16.1). Given the appropriate return to hemodynamic baseline in combination with normal lab values, the decision was made to proceed with the case, which was completed without further incident. The patient was recovered and kept overnight for observation with cardiac monitoring – he was ultimately discharged to home the following day in stable condition. The patient was subsequently seen in follow-up 1 week postoperatively, at which time he was doing well with no evidence of turbinate necrosis or other postoperative sequelae from the errant injection.

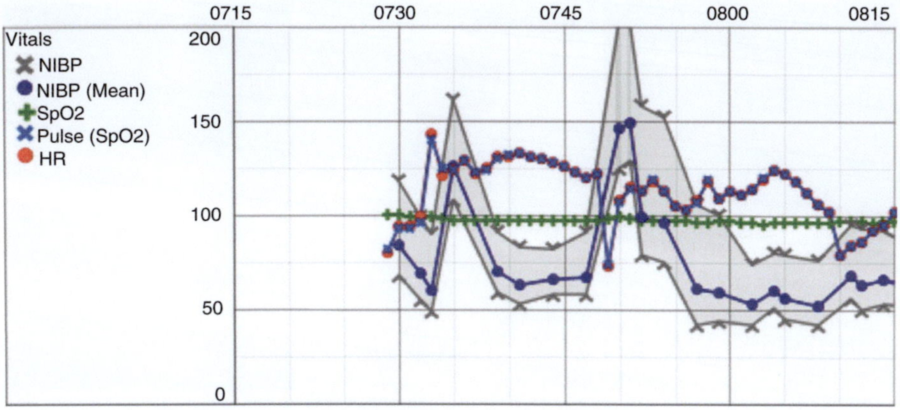

Fig. 16.1 Intraoperative blood pressure changes, as represented by the anesthesia machine. Note the expected rise in blood pressure (NIBP) upon induction, followed by a more dramatic spike minutes later representing the errant infusion of concentrated epinephrine

While this situation did not ultimately result in any significant immediate or long-term adverse consequences, it highlights the critical importance of appropriately identifying and labeling all injectable solutions in the operating room. This chapter discusses the various uses of epinephrine in the hospital setting, particularly within the operating room, as well as common pitfalls with its use and potential methods to avoid them.

Root Cause Analysis

Several independent permissive factors were identified that contributed to the described situation. First, general safety practices (and often institutional policies) dictate that 1:1000 epinephrine be dispensed into a separate container, together with fluorescein, to clearly differentiate this solution from any injectable concentration of epinephrine containing local anesthetic. Additionally, best practices would suggest that any solution being drawn up into a syringe should be pre-labeled or labeled immediately to avoid confusion [1]. Unfortunately, neither of these practices was followed in this event.

From a distribution safety standpoint, the particular epinephrine product used (1:1000 epinephrine) was contained in a 30 mL glass container with a magenta cap that is similar in appearance to the bottle containing 1% lidocaine with 1:100,000 epinephrine, one of the more commonly used intraoperative injectable solutions (Fig. 16.2). Additionally, this solution comes in a vial that necessitates a syringe to access, as opposed to other formulations that are available in breakable ampules that can then be dispensed directly into an open container. This necessitates that even

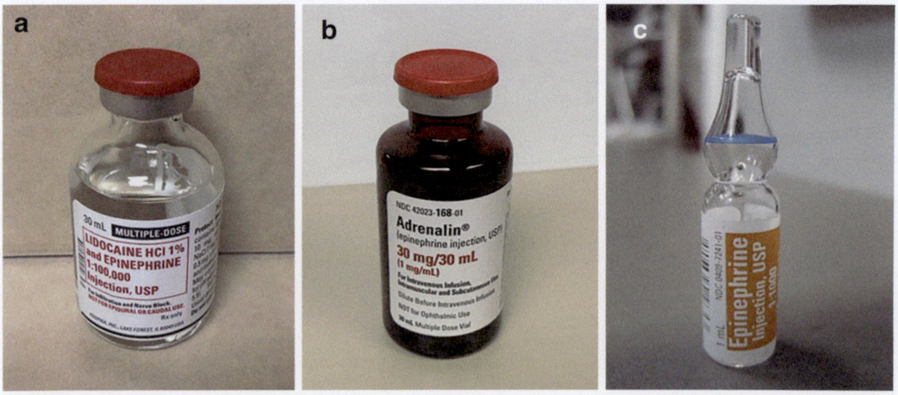

Fig. 16.2 (**a**) Lidocaine 1% with 1:100,000 epinephrine. (**b**) Adrenalin® 1 mg/mL. (**c**) Epinephrine 1:1000 single-use ampule. Note the similarities in shape, size and color-coding of cap and label, as well as the inconsistencies in concentration labeling

when extreme caution is used, there will always be a point in the process during which concentrated epinephrine is contained in a syringe, creating an opportunity for error.

Lessons Learned

An understanding of the pharmacology and physiologic effects of epinephrine is critical. Epinephrine or adrenaline, a nonselective agonist of alpha-1, alpha-2, beta-1, and beta-2 receptors has a broad list of indications within the hospital setting, both inside and outside of the operating room. These include anaphylactic reactions, bronchospasm, shock and cardiac arrest, among others [2] (Table 16.1). Clinically applicable dosages of epinephrine are frequently indicated in milligrams, while distributed volumes are classically labeled with concentration ratios of grams per milliliter. There is, however, a disconnect between how these concentrations are viewed by pharmacists and non-pharmacists, leading to an ongoing change in the labeling system for epinephrine – labels are now suggested to list mass concentration rather than simple ratios. For example, 1:1000 epinephrine (the concentration commonly used *topically* in nasal and sinus surgery) is now labeled as 1 mg/mL, while 1:10,000 epinephrine (the IV concentration used in cardiac arrest) is now labeled 0.1 mg/mL.

The primary reasons for this change include an attempt to reduce calculation errors, and a shift in focus to clinical application rather than pharmaceutical techniques for mixing solutions. While these calculations on paper may seem straightforward, requiring healthcare providers to make conversions during potentially life-threatening situations creates the very real potential for error. A study by Rolf and Harper, which surveyed physicians from 150 teaching hospitals in Great Britain,

Table 16.1 Common epinephrine dosing in otolaryngology [3]

Use		Dose
Topical	Adults:	1:1000 (1 mg/mL) epinephrine intranasal, on cotton pledgets
	Pediatrics:	Avoid if able; 1:2000 (0.5 mg/mL) epinephrine intranasal, on cotton pledgets
	Frequency:	As needed
Local anesthesia adjunct	Adults:	1:200,000 (0.005 mg/mL) to 1:50,000 (0.02 mg/mL) epinephrine SC
	Pediatrics:	1:200,000 (0.005 mg/mL) to 1:50,000 (0.02 mg/mL) epinephrine SC
	Frequency:	Per duration of added anesthestic
Bronchospasm	Adults:	0.3–0.5 mg of 1:1000 (1 mg/mL) epinephrine SC
	Pediatrics:	0.01 mg/kg of 1:1000 (1 mg/mL) epinephrine SC in children <30 kg
	Frequency:	Every 20 minutes for three doses
Anaphylaxis	Adults:	0.3–0.5 mg of 1:1000 (1 mg/mL) epinephrine IM
	Pediatrics:	0.01 mg/kg of 1:1000 (1 mg/mL) epinephrine IM in children <30 kg
	Frequency:	Every 5–10 minutes as needed
Cardiac arrest	Adults:	0.5–1.0 mg of 1:10,000 (0.1 mg/mL) epinephrine IV
	Pediatrics:	0.01 mg/kg of 1:10,000 (0.1 mg/mL) epinephrine IV in children <50 kg
	Frequency:	Every 3–5 minutes as needed; Do not interrupt CPR to administer
Shock	Adults:	0.1 mcg/kg/min of 1:1,000,000 (1 mcg/mL) epinephrine, continuous IV infusion
	Pediatrics:	0.1 mcg/kg/min of 1:100,000 (10 mcg/mL) epinephrine, continuous IV infusion
	Frequency:	Titrate every 2–3 minutes in increments of 0.05 mcg/kg/min to desired MAP

SC subcutaneous, *IM* intramuscular, *IV* intravenous, *CPR* cardiopulmonary resuscitation, *MAP* mean arterial pressure

demonstrated that over 40% of physicians were unable to consistently convert drug dosages correctly in a controlled situation [4]. Likewise, a randomized trial conducted in a simulation setting demonstrated that physicians were more prone to over-administer epinephrine, and took over 1.5 minutes longer to do so, when using ratios rather than mass concentrations [5]. To decrease the need for these types of calculations during practice in real-time, many hospitals now stock individual injection dosages in crash carts for high-acuity scenarios (e.g., 1:1000 [1 mg/mL] epinephrine in an anaphylaxis kit) [6].

While these types of institutional changes are beneficial for clinical situations with clear indications such as anaphylaxis or cardiac arrest, uses and dosages of epinephrine can vary widely in the surgical setting. In the operating room, several different dilutions of epinephrine are routinely used, either alone for topical hemostasis or in combination with local anesthetic injections. The benefits of epinephrine in the latter capacity are twofold: it restricts vascular absorption, which modifies the duration of anesthetic effect, and encourages vasoconstriction, which improves intraoperative hemostasis. In situations where epinephrine is combined with a local anesthetic, the maximal dose is typically limited by that of the local anesthetic (Table 16.2). Studies have demonstrated that when combined with a local anesthetic, concentrations of epinephrine between 1:400,000 (0.0025 mg/mL) and 1:100,000 (0.01 mg/mL) are equally effective in achieving the desired vasoconstrictive effects, while providing a proportional increase in duration of action [7]. Often more than one different concentration of local anesthetic and/or epinephrine are used within the same case, making clear identification of each concentration vital to patient safety.

Topical 1:1000 (1 mg/mL) epinephrine is frequently used as a decongestant to achieve hemostasis and improve visualization during endonasal and endoscopic sinus surgery. This role was historically filled by 4% cocaine (a combination sodium channel blocker and serotonin-norepinephrine-dopamine reuptake inhibitor [SNDRI]), which has largely been abandoned due to its unpredictable cardiovascular impact and its physiologic potentiation of excitatory effects caused by injectable epinephrine [9]. Another common alternative is oxymetazoline (a selective alpha-1 and partial alpha-2 agonist), which has a more favorable safety profile but less potent vasoconstrictive effects. A number of studies have shown that topical epinephrine achieves equivalent visualization and hemostasis to that of cocaine [9, 10], while maintaining an acceptable systemic profile more akin to that of oxymetazoline [11, 12]. Intranasal infiltration of dilute epinephrine (1:100,000 [1 mg/mL]) to induce local vasoconstriction has been suggested as a strategy to mitigate the systemic absorption of topical epinephrine [13] – while this may limit the hemodynamic impact of topical epinephrine, it does carry the added risk of inadvertent intravascular injection [14]. Best practices in otolaryngology indicate that each of the above strategies is safe for use in endonasal and endoscopic sinus surgery, which

Table 16.2 Maximum recommended doses for infiltration of commonly used local anesthetics in otolaryngology [8]

		Max dose by weight (mg/kg)		Absolute max dose (mg)
Drug	Typical concentration	Plain	w/epinephrine	Plain/+epi
Esters				
Procaine	1%	7.0	10.0	800/1000
Chloroprocaine	1%	10.0	14.0	800/1000
Amides				
Bupivacaine	0.25%	2.0	3.0	175/225
Lidocaine	0.5%, 1%, 2%	4.5	7.0	300/500
Mepivacaine	0.5%, 1%	4.5	6.6	400/500
Ropivacaine	0.2%, 0.5%	3.0	4.0	200

again illustrates the importance of appropriate drug identification to avoid negligent errors.

Though epinephrine overdose is a common topic in the literature, there is no clearly defined maximum dose of systemic epinephrine. While it has been suggested that the minimal lethal dose of *subcutaneous* epinephrine exceeds several milligrams, undesirable local and systemic reactions occur at much lower doses [15]. In the awake patient, symptoms of toxicity can initially present as headache, dizziness, nausea, palpitations, tremor, and generalized weakness. Signs of progressive toxicity include systemic and intracranial hypertension, wheezing or bronchospasm, and cardiac arrhythmias [16]. There have even been several published case reports documenting acute myocardial infarction following intramuscular (IM) administration of epinephrine in the setting of anaphylaxis [17]. In the operating room, anticipated hemodynamic changes would include hypertension, tachycardia, and arrhythmias, along with electrolyte disturbances including hypokalemia and lactic acidosis. Readily apparent to the surgeon would be early signs of local tissue ischemia followed by subsequent necrosis, which should certainly raise suspicion for local epinephrine toxicity [16].

The treatment of systemic epinephrine toxicity should be directed at hemodynamic control, with a particular emphasis on blood pressure regulation to avoid myocardial ischemia and intracerebral hemorrhage. The inherent beta agonism of epinephrine causes increased heart rate and cardiac contractility that may lead to potentially lethal arrhythmias. Likewise, alpha receptor stimulation leads to increased systemic vascular resistance and thus increased afterload on the heart [18]. As such, it is important to avoid pure beta blockade in treating epinephrine toxicity as it will acutely weaken cardiac contractility and can precipitate pulmonary edema and ultimately cardiovascular collapse. Labetalol, a mixed alpha/beta antagonist, or phentolamine, a nonselective alpha antagonist are reasonable choices for acute symptomatic management. Nitric oxide derivatives (e.g., Nitroglycerine), calcium channel blockers, or Propofol are preferred for their vasodilatory and cardiac contractility effects independent of the catecholamine pathway [19].

Fortunately, lasting adverse outcomes were avoided in the reported case. It does, however, highlight the critical nature of mixing and dispensing medications in the OR setting. This is also not a new or unique issue – a recent survey of practicing otolaryngologists demonstrated that over one-fourth of respondents had experienced or heard of misadministration of concentrated epinephrine occurring during the previous year [20]. This further emphasizes the importance of rigorous hospital protocols regarding injectable solutions – notably immediate labeling and dispensing of epinephrine into a container with fluorescein for topical use to differentiate it from other injectable solutions. If either of these practices had been properly followed, the event in the presented case, and many others like it, may have been prevented entirely.

Outside of meticulous labeling and judicious division of injectable solutions on the operative field, several other precautions can be taken to avoid such errors. Hospitals can work to store a single concentration of epinephrine wherever possible, and the pharmacy can be relied upon to prepare concentrated epinephrine if

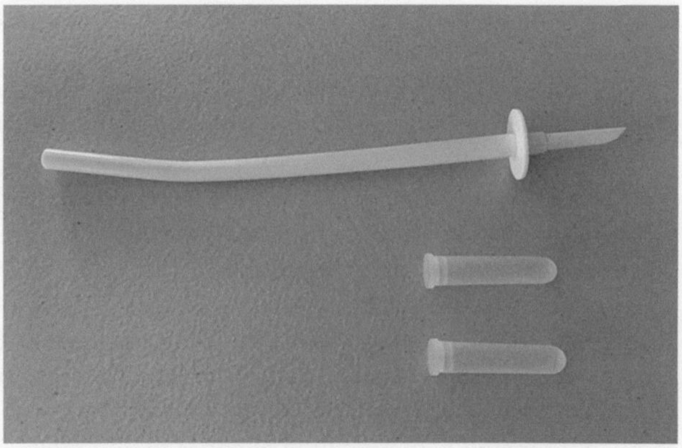

Fig. 16.3 Vial decanter for aseptic transfer of fluids. Sharp end is used to penetrate the septum of a vial, allowing for sterile contents to be poured directly into an alternate vessel for easy access without the need for a syringe

needed. Likewise, a change from vials to breakable ampules, or the use of vial decanters (Fig. 16.3) could avoid the need to draw concentrated epinephrine into a syringe entirely. As always, communication is vital – both in clearly acknowledging when injectable substances are exchanged between personnel, and in verifying concentrations prior to injection. Finally, while pharmaceutical companies work to express drugs exclusively as mass concentrations, they should consider implementation of complementary colored labels or different colored solutions to easily distinguish commonly injectable solutions. While implementation of safety net protocols like those suggested here can help to reduce errors, it is ultimately up to the surgeon and the entire operative team to remain vigilant throughout any case where injectable medications are used.

References

1. Kuan EC, Tajudeen BA, Bhandarkar ND, St John MA, Palmer JN, Adappa ND. Is topical epinephrine safe for hemostasis in endoscopic sinus surgery? Laryngoscope. 2019;129(1):1–3. https://doi.org/10.1002/lary.27238.
2. Epinephrine Injection [Internet]. MedlinePlus. U.S. National Library of Medicine. Available from: https://medlineplus.gov/druginfo/meds/a603002.html.
3. Epinephrine [Internet]. PubChem compound database. U.S. National Library of Medicine. Available from: https://pubchem.ncbi.nlm.nih.gov/compound/5816#section=Pharmacology.
4. Rolfe S, Harper NJ. Ability of hospital doctors to calculate drug doses. BMJ. 1995;310(6988):1173–4. https://doi.org/10.1136/bmj.310.6988.1173.
5. Wheeler DW, Carter JJ, Murray LJ, Degnan BA, Dunling CP, Salvador R, Menon DK, Gupta AK. The effect of drug concentration expression on epinephrine dosing errors: a randomized trial. Ann Intern Med. 2008;148(1):11–4. https://doi.org/10.7326/0003-4819-148-1-200801010-00003.
6. Kanwar M, Irvin CB, Frank JJ, Weber K, Rosman H. Confusion about epinephrine dosing leading to iatrogenic overdose: a life-threatening problem with a potential solution. Ann Emerg Med. 2010;55(4):341–4. https://doi.org/10.1016/j.annemergmed.2009.11.008.

7. Kim H, Hwang K, Yun SM, Kim DJ. Usage of epinephrine mixed with lidocaine in plastic surgery. J Craniofac Surg. 2020;31(3):791–3. https://doi.org/10.1097/SCS.0000000000006156.
8. Malamed SF. Handbook of local anesthesia. 7th ed. Edinburg: Elsevier; 2020. ISBN-13: 978-0323582070.
9. Valdes CJ, Bogado M, Rammal A, Samaha M, Tewfik MA. Topical cocaine vs adrenaline in endoscopic sinus surgery: a blinded randomized controlled study. Int Forum Allergy Rhinol. 2014;4(8):646–50. https://doi.org/10.1002/alr.21325.
10. Ahmed OG, Yu J, Choi JS, Yim MT, Yoshor D, Takashima M. Real-time hemodynamic effects of 1:100,000 and 1:200,000 injectable epinephrine and placement of topical 1:1000 epinephrine pledgets in patients undergoing endoscopic sinus and skull-base surgery: a randomized, prospective study. Int Forum Allergy Rhinol. 2020;10(2):141–6. https://doi.org/10.1002/alr.22493.
11. Korkmaz H, Yao WC, Korkmaz M, Bleier BS. Safety and efficacy of concentrated topical epinephrine use in endoscopic endonasal surgery. Int Forum Allergy Rhinol. 2015;5(12):1118–23. https://doi.org/10.1002/alr.21590.
12. Yim MT, Ahmed OG, Takashima M. Evaluating real-time effects of topical 1:1000 epinephrine in endoscopic sinus and skull-base surgery on hemodynamic parameters through intraoperative arterial line monitoring. Int Forum Allergy Rhinol. 2017;7(11):1065–9. https://doi.org/10.1002/alr.22012.
13. Gunaratne DA, Barham HP, Christensen JM, Bhatia DD, Stamm AC, Harvey RJ. Topical concentrated epinephrine (1:1000) does not cause acute cardiovascular changes during endoscopic sinus surgery. Int Forum Allergy Rhinol. 2016;6(2):135–9. https://doi.org/10.1002/alr.21642.
14. Kennedy DW. Management of the visual field in endoscopic sinus surgery. Int Forum Allergy Rhinol. 2020;10(2):139–40. https://doi.org/10.1002/alr.22527.
15. Fernando DM, Dayaratne KM. Adrenaline toxicity following accidental administration of the 1:1000 solution during dental procedures: four case reports. J Forensic Legal Med. 2012;19(5):302–4. https://doi.org/10.1016/j.jflm.2012.02.015.
16. Adrenalin® (Epinephrine injection) [package insert on the Internet]. Mukilteo, WA: HF Acquisition Co. LLC, DBA HealthFirst. [Revised Feb 2020]. Available from: https://nctr-crs.fda.gov/fdalabel/services/spl/set-ids/7663c49d-1b1d-755d-e053-2991aa0a4ee3/spl-doc?hl=adrenalin.
17. Jayamali WD, Herath HMMTB, Kulathunga A. Myocardial infarction during anaphylaxis in a young healthy male with normal coronary arteries- is epinephrine the culprit? BMC Cardiovasc Disord. 2017;17(1):237. https://doi.org/10.1186/s12872-017-0670-7.
18. Overgaard CB, Dzavík V. Inotropes and vasopressors: review of physiology and clinical use in cardiovascular disease. Circulation. 2008;118(10):1047–56. https://doi.org/10.1161/CIRCULATIONAHA.107.728840.
19. Mathez C, Favrat B, Staeger P. Management options for accidental injection of epinephrine from an autoinjector: a case report. J Med Case Rep. 2009;3:7268. https://doi.org/10.4076/1752-1947-3-7268.
20. Shah RK, Hoy E, Roberson DW, Nielsen D. Errors with concentrated epinephrine in otolaryngology. Laryngoscope. 2008;118(11):1928–30. https://doi.org/10.1097/MLG.0b013e318180ec.

Chapter 17
Bleeding in FESS

Ashton E. Lehmann and Benjamin S. Bleier

Clinical Pearls

1. Bleeding during FESS can obscure the surgical field, leading to poor visualization of critical anatomic areas, thereby increasing complication risk.
2. Optimization of hemostasis in FESS requires preoperative planning, including review of preoperative medications and choice of anesthetic technique.
3. Intraoperative considerations include Trendelenburg positioning and use of concentrated epinephrine with appropriate safety protocols to avoid inadvertent injection.

Case Report

A 63-year-old woman with chronic rhinosinusitis (CRS) with nasal polyps is recovering in the PACU from a functional endoscopic sinus surgery (FESS). While straining, she has brisk left-sided epistaxis, unresponsive to pressure and only slightly attenuated with thrombin-gelatin hemostatic matrix (Surgiflo). She then has rapid

Supplementary Information The online version of this chapter (https://doi.org/10.1007/978-3-030-75323-8_17) contains supplementary material, which is available to authorized users.

A. E. Lehmann (✉)
Department of Otolaryngology–Head and Neck Surgery, Vanderbilt University Medical Center, Nashville, TN, USA
e-mail: ashton.lehmann@vumc.org

B. S. Bleier
Department of Otolaryngology, Massachusetts Eye and Ear Infirmary, Harvard Medical School, Boston, MA, USA

R. K. Chandra, K. C. Welch (eds.), *Lessons Learned from Rhinologic Procedure Complications*, https://doi.org/10.1007/978-3-030-75323-8_17

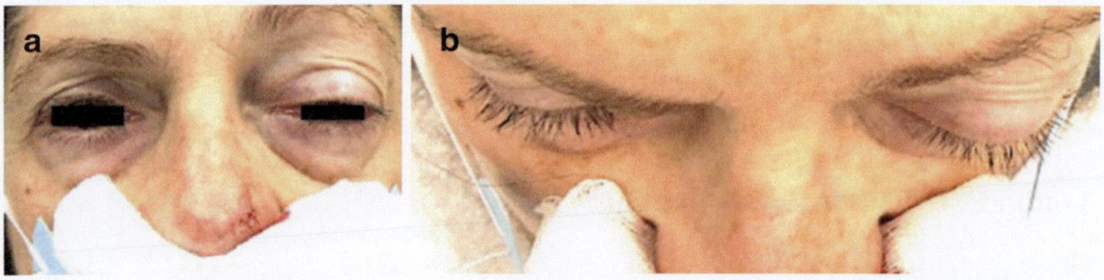

Fig. 17.1 A patient with CRS with nasal polyps post-FESS in the PACU has left-sided epistaxis and proptosis, with decreased visual acuity and elevated intraocular pressure, raising concern for a retrobulbar hematoma. (**a**) Frontal view in PACU. (**b**) Bird's eye view in PACU

onset of ipsilateral proptosis with inability to fully open her left eyelid (Fig. 17.1). The rhinology and ophthalmology teams are emergently consulted. The surgeon reports that the FESS was uneventful aside from extensive polyposis and being rather bloody, especially when dissecting the left frontal ostium. The bleeding substantially slowed by the end of the case and no packing was placed.

On examination, the patient's left-sided visual acuity has decreased and the intraocular pressure (IOP) is elevated to 31 mmHg. The history and exam findings raise concern for orbital compartment syndrome due to a rapidly expanding retrobulbar hematoma, likely from an anterior ethmoid artery (AEA) injury with retraction into the orbit. If packing had been in place, this would be removed to decrease unnecessary pressure on the orbit. As plans are made to emergently return to the operating room (OR) for definitive management, the globe becomes increasingly tense and the IOP rises to 51 mmHg within moments. A lateral canthotomy and inferior cantholysis are completed emergently (*accompanying example video of lateral canthotomy/inferior cantholysis available online* (Video 17.1)). This maneuver is indicated based upon the clinical findings regardless of whether IOP measurement is available.

As the patient returns to the OR, avenues for AEA bleeding management are considered, including the transcaruncular, endoscopic endonasal, and endoscopic intraorbital approaches (*accompanying example video of each of these approaches available online* (Videos 17.2, 17.3, and 17.4)). As endoscopic equipment is readily available, and there is need to control epistaxis, intraorbital AEA bleeding, and IOP, the endoscopic endonasal/intraorbital approach is chosen. This is completed with further orbital decompression and good control of bleeding in both the nose and orbit. Postoperatively, the IOP normalizes to 17 mmHg and the visual acuity returns to baseline. At follow-up 1 week later, the patient is recovering without further incident, and the canthotomy/cantholysis is healing well by secondary intention.

Root Cause Analysis

A retrobulbar hematoma is a dreaded complication of FESS. In reviewing the case that preceded this complication, the original FESS was noted to be bloody. Bleeding during FESS can obscure the surgical field, leading to poor visualization of critical anatomic areas, thereby increasing the risk of complications [1]. Bleeding intraoperatively, as well as altered or obscured anatomy due to extensive nasal polyposis, could have increased the risk of untoward and even unrecognized damage to structures in the above case, such as the AEA [2]. Following AEA violation, the vessel can spasm and subsequently bleed in a delayed fashion. Conversely, apparent cessation of bleeding may lessen the surgeon's concern for a complication, when all the while the artery has retracted into the orbit creating an evolving retrobulbar hematoma. This complication could perhaps have been prevented with improved hemostasis and visualization during the original FESS. Hemostasis can be optimized with proper preoperative planning, effective surgical field preparation, and consideration of surgical technique.

Lessons Learned

Hemostatic Preoperative Planning

Optimal hemostasis in FESS starts in advance of the surgery. Based on reported data from 6852 surgical patients in the United States, 34% of patients report having taken in the 2 weeks leading up to surgery complementary and alternative medicines that may potentially inhibit coagulation [3]. These reported medicines include bromelain, borage, cayenne, celery, chamomile, dandelion, dong quai, evening primrose, fenugreek, feverfew, fish oil, garlic, ginger, ginkgo, ginseng, hawthorn, horse chestnut, huang qi, kava kava, licorice, papain, red clover, turmeric, and vitamin E [3]. Given the additional bleeding risk they pose, such medicines should be stopped at least 10 days preoperatively [2].

In patients with CRS with nasal polyps, preoperative steroid treatment appears to reduce operative blood loss (OBL). In a double-blinded, randomized, placebo-controlled study of 23 patients with severe nasal polyps undergoing FESS, Ecevit et al. found that preoperative oral steroids (prednisolone for 2 weeks) improve surgical field visibility ($p = 0.003$) and reduce OBL (141 ± 90 versus 384.2 ± 237.5 mL, $p = 0.022$) without a significant increase in complication rate ($p = 0.214$) compared to placebo [4]. This beneficial effect of steroids is not observed in patients with CRS without nasal polyps [5], and it may depend upon the duration of steroid course employed in patients with nasal polyps. In a surgeon-blinded, randomized trial of 80 patients with CRS with nasal polyps, Atighechi et al. found a five-day preoperative prednisolone course significantly reduced OBL compared to a single steroid dose the day before surgery (206 ± 52.81 vs. 266.5 ± 96.31 mL, $p = 0.038$), despite similar mean arterial pressure (MAP) readings in both groups (70–80 mmHg) [6].

Optimizing hemostasis in FESS also requires advanced planning with the anesthesia team to optimize anesthetic and hemodynamic conditions. High-quality evidence has demonstrated that total intravenous anesthesia (TIVA) improves surgical field visibility compared to inhalational techniques [7]. In a prospective, randomized, controlled trial of 56 patients undergoing FESS, Wormald et al. found TIVA (propofol with a remifentanil infusion) compared to inhalation anesthesia (sevoflurane with incremental fentanyl doses) offered significantly better surgical field quality ($p < 0.001$) [1]. In this study, the MAP ($p = 0.003$) and pulse ($p = 0.036$) independently influenced surgical field quality, suggesting that maintenance of lower MAP and pulse also improves surgical field visibility [1]. The anesthetic plans and hemodynamic goals should be discussed between the surgical and anesthesia teams before the start of the case to ensure agreement.

Hemostatic Surgical Field Preparation

Following induction, choices regarding patient positioning, topical vasoconstriction, and local injection all influence hemostasis during FESS. In a prospective, randomized controlled trial of 64 patients with CRS undergoing FESS, Hathorn et al. found 15° reverse Trendelenburg positioning compared to horizontal positioning decreased OBL ($p = 0.01$) and improved surgical field visibility ($p < 0.001$) despite similar MAP readings in both groups ($p > 0.05$) [8].

Despite widespread use of either oxymetazoline, phenylephrine, or cocaine for topical vasoconstriction, in a systematic review of 20 articles exploring bleeding control in FESS, Valiente et al. found no sufficiently strong evidence to suggest these agents are more effective compared to others or placebo in decreasing OBL or improving visibility [9]. Moderate quality evidence, however, suggests that topical application of concentrated epinephrine is effective at the 1:2000 concentration and safe even at the 1:1000 concentration [7]. In a prospective, double-blinded, randomized trial of 49 patients undergoing FESS, Sarmento et al. compared different topical epinephrine concentrations (i.e., 1:2000, 1:10,000, and 1:50,000) and found significantly less OBL in the 1:2000 group ($p < 0.0001$) [10].

Multiple studies have supported the safety of topical concentrated epinephrine. A retrospective review of 1140 patients receiving intranasal topical 1:1000 epinephrine found no intraoperative cardiovascular complications and no elevated risk of postoperative rebound epistaxis [11]. In a larger retrospective review of 1998 patients undergoing FESS with topical 1:1000 epinephrine usage, Orlandi et al. found a complication rate of only 0.1% attributable to concentrated epinephrine: one case of coronary artery vasospasm and one case of transient intraoperative hypertension immediately following inadvertent submucosal injection of 1:1000 epinephrine (accidentally switched with 1% lidocaine/1:100,000 epinephrine) [12]. Preventative safeguards (e.g., instillation of a drop of methylene blue or fluorescein to differentiate the topical concentrated epinephrine from injectable concentrations) can be employed to decrease the risk of inadvertent injection. In a series of 26 patients undergoing endoscopic transsphenoidal surgery, Yim et al. utilized arterial line readings to monitor the hemodynamic effects of topical 1:1000 epinephrine-soaked pledgets placed intranasally: There were no intraoperative or postoperative complications attributed to the concentrated epinephrine usage, but 23% of patients had significant transient increases in blood pressure, some of which required medical intervention to return to baseline [13]. Thus, the potential for complication exists when concentrated epinephrine is used; however, with appropriate safeguards and special consideration of at-risk patient populations (e.g., patients with elevated cardiac risk), topical concentrated epinephrine use is safe in FESS [12, 13].

Moderate quality evidence also suggests injection of epinephrine containing local anesthetic solution improves surgical field visibility [7]. In a double-blinded, randomized controlled trial of 22 patients undergoing endoscopic nasal surgery comparing injection of 1% lidocaine/1:100,000 epinephrine to injection of saline alone, the surgeons reported bloodier surgical fields in the saline-injected patients ($p < 0.05$) despite use of topical 1:1000 epinephrine-soaked pledgets in both groups [14].

Some studies, however, have raised safety concerns depending on the concentration of epinephrine injected. In a double-blinded, randomized trial of 140 patients undergoing FESS, Moshaver et al. found significant hemodynamic fluctuations (i.e., increased pulse, blood pressure, and MAP) following submucosal injection of 2% lidocaine/1:100,000 epinephrine ($p > 0.05$ for all) but not following injection of 2% lidocaine/1:200,000 epinephrine [15]. The authors found no difference in OBL between the epinephrine concentrations ($p > 0.05$), leading them to conclude that local injection of 2% lidocaine/1:200,000 epinephrine avoids hemodynamic fluctuations while offering a similar hemostatic profile as local injection of 2% lidocaine/1:100,000 [15]. In a case-control study of 452 patients with bilateral CRS undergoing FESS, Lee et al. compared submucosal injections of 1:100,000 epinephrine to topical application of 1:100,000 epinephrine: No significant difference in OBL was observed between the injection group and the topical group (316.9 ± 162.1 vs. 333.9 ± 167.8 mL, $p = 0.29$), but there was a higher rate of transient cardiac dysrhythmias in the injection group (21% vs. 0%, $p < 0.001$) [16]. The authors concluded it may be advisable to avoid local injection of 1:100,000 epinephrine during FESS without increased OBL compared to topical 1:100,000 epinephrine usage [16]. These results suggest that local injection may provide enhanced hemostasis compared to topical vasoconstriction alone, but significant hemodynamic and cardiac risks may exist when 1:100,000 epinephrine is injected during FESS.

Hemostatic Operative Techniques

Numerous surgical techniques may be practiced to minimize unwanted bleeding during FESS. Atraumatic placement of the endoscope and instruments and atraumatic suction usage can avoid unwanted mucosal injury [2]. Use of sharp dissection with through-biting or through-cutting instrumentation or microdebriders decreases the risk of pulling or stripping mucosa, which can result in unwanted bleeding [2]. A methodical surgical approach with efficient debulking of inflammatory tissue (e.g., nasal polyps) and progression from inferior to superior in the field when able can also minimize bleeding [2]. Establishing surgical landmarks intraoperatively enables appropriate caution around higher risk areas for bleeding complications due to vascular injury [2]. And in cases of nasal polyps, the initial application of vasoconstricting agents may be restricted due to compromised visualization from the polyps. Thus, as the inflammatory disease is debulked, further application of vasoconstricting agents to newly visualized tissue may be indicated [2].

When bleeding is encountered during FESS, identification of the source of bleeding (e.g., mucosa, bone, or a named vessel) is critical [2]. Persistent oozing may obscure the field and render it more difficult or impossible to trace prominent bleeding to a specific source [2]. Replacement of topical vasoconstricting agents on surgical pledgets, warm (49 °C) saline bulb irrigations, or communication with the anesthesia team to optimize hemodynamic parameters may help when surgical field visibility is compromised by bleeding [2]. If bone bleeding is encountered, hemostatic material may be placed over the bleeding site (and pressure gently applied with a pledget) or a diamond burr may be used to physically occlude the bleeding bone site [2].

Cauterization of specific bleeding sites with monopolar or bipolar cautery is at times indicated [2]. For FESS, cautery apparatus should be present in the room and tested preoperatively, the patient should be grounded at the start of the case, and the cautery pedals should be readily accessible to the surgeon in case cautery is needed expeditiously. Brisk, rapid-onset bleeding suggests inadvertent vascular injury and merits identification and control of the bleeding source [2]. Detailed hemostatic control of injured named vessels is reviewed in other chapters of this text.

During FESS, it is imperative to expose and identify any persistent bleeding areas. Obscuring blood staining or clots may be washed away with irrigations. High-risk bleeding areas should be checked for hemostasis (e.g., posterior septal artery territory around the sphenoid rostrum, sphenopalatine artery territory, and roots of the middle and inferior turbinates). Hemostasis may be further confirmed with a Valsalva maneuver provided by the anesthesia team [2]. Only once bleeding has been controlled and hemostasis confirmed should emergence from anesthesia be considered.

Hemostatic Packing Considerations

Hemostatic packing may be considered in select cases when alternative hemostatic interventions (e.g., cautery) are not indicated. In a review of the literature of middle meatal dressings available for use at the end of FESS, Soler and Schlosser concluded that level 1 evidence exists to support the use of chitosan, gelatin granules combined with human thrombin (Floseal), or microporous polysaccharide hemospheres (MPH, Medafor) to improve perioperative hemostasis, but no studies demonstrate improvement in postoperative hemorrhage rates [17].

Among these dressings, only chitosan also has level 1 evidence of reduced synechiae formation [17]. In a randomized controlled trial of 40 patients with CRS undergoing FESS with unilateral chitosan gel packing (without any contralateral packing), Valentine et al. found chitosan gel demonstrated rapid hemostasis (within

2 min on average) compared to the control side without packing (10 min on average, $p < 0.001$), as well as significantly less adhesions up to 12 weeks postoperatively ($p < 0.001$) [18].

In summary, bleeding during FESS may compromise visualization, thereby increasing complication risk [1, 2]. Optimizing hemostasis in FESS involves preoperative planning, surgical field preparation, specific operative techniques, and selective use of hemostatic packing. Only with adequate hemostasis in FESS may the surgical field visibility be sufficient to achieve surgical goals without increased risk [2].

References

1. Wormald PJ, van Renen G, Perks J, Jones JA, Langton-Hewer CD. The effect of the total intravenous anesthesia compared with inhalational anesthesia on the surgical field during endoscopic sinus surgery. Am J Rhinol. 2005;19(5):514–20.
2. Pant H. Hemostasis in endoscopic sinus surgery. Otolaryngol Clin N Am. 2016;49(3):655–76.
3. Norred CL. Complementary and alternative medicine use by surgical patients. AORN J. 2002;76(6):1013–21.
4. Ecevit MC, Erdag TK, Dogan E, Sutay S. Effect of steroids for nasal polyposis surgery: a placebo-controlled, randomized, double-blind study. Laryngoscope. 2015;125(9):2041–5.
5. Fraire ME, Sanchez-Vallecillo MV, Zernotti ME, Paoletti OA. Effect of premedication with systemic steroids on surgical field bleeding and visibility during nasosinusal endoscopic surgery. Acta Otorrinolaringol Esp. 2013;64(2):133–9.
6. Atighechi S, Azimi MR, Mirvakili SA, Baradaranfar MH, Dadgarnia MH. Evaluation of intraoperative bleeding during an endoscopic surgery of nasal polyposis after a preoperative single dose versus a 5-day course of corticosteroid. Eur Arch Otorhinolaryngol. 2013;270(9):2451–4.
7. Timperley D. Perioperative bleeding and vascular control. In: Schlosser RJ, Harvey RJ, editors. Endoscopic sinus surgery: optimizing outcomes and avoiding failures. San Diego: Plural Publishing; 2012.
8. Hathorn IF, Habib A-RR, Manji J, Javer AR. Comparing the reverse Trendelenburg and horizontal position for endoscopic sinus surgery: a randomized controlled trial. Otolaryngol Head Neck Surg. 2013;148(2):308–13.
9. Rodriguez Valiente A, Roldan Fidalgo A, Laguna Ortega D. Bleeding control in endoscopic sinus surgery: a systematic review of the literature. Rhinology. 2013;51(4):298–305.
10. de Araujo Sarmento KM, Tomita S, de Avila Kós AO. Topical use of adrenaline in different concentrations for endoscopic sinus surgery. Braz J Otorhinolaryngol. 2009;75(2):280–9.
11. Korkmaz H, Yao WC, Korkmaz M, Bleier BS. Safety and efficacy of concentrated topical epinephrine use in endoscopic endonasal surgery. Int Forum Allergy Rhinol. 2015;5(12):1118–23.
12. Orlandi RR, Warrier S, Sato S, Han JK. Concentrated topical epinephrine is safe in endoscopic sinus surgery. Am J Rhinol Allergy. 2010;24(2):140–2.
13. Yim MT, Ahmed OG, Takashima M. Evaluating real-time effects of topical 1:1000 epinephrine in endoscopic sinus and skull-base surgery on hemodynamic parameters through intraoperative arterial line monitoring. Int Forum Allergy Rhinol. 2017;7(11):1065–9.
14. Cohen-Kerem R, Brown S, Villaseñor LV, Witterick I. Epinephrine/lidocaine injection vs. saline during endoscopic sinus surgery. Laryngoscope. 2008;118(7):1275–81.
15. Moshaver A, Lin D, Pinto R, Witterick IJ. The hemostatic and hemodynamic effects of epinephrine during endoscopic sinus surgery: a randomized clinical trial. Arch Otolaryngol Head Neck Surg. 2009;135(10):1005–9.

16. Lee T-J, Huang C-C, Chang P-H, Chang C-J, Chen Y-W. Hemostasis during functional endoscopic sinus surgery: the effect of local infiltration with adrenaline. Otolaryngol Head Neck Surg. 2009;140(2):209–14.
17. Soler ZM, Schlosser RJ. Post-FESS middle meatal dressings: avoiding the inevitable? JAMA Otolaryngol Head Neck Surg. 2013;139(12):1351–4.
18. Valentine R, Athanasiadis T, Moratti S, Hanton L, Robinson S, Wormald P-J. The efficacy of a novel chitosan gel on hemostasis and wound healing after endoscopic sinus surgery. Am J Rhinol Allergy. 2010;24(1):70–5.

Chapter 18
Sphenopalatine Artery Bleeding from Maxillary Mega-Antrostomy

Conner J. Massey and Vijay R. Ramakrishnan

Clinical Pearls

1. The sphenopalatine artery has two branches that supply the posterior nasal cavity: the posterior lateral nasal branch, which supplies the lateral nasal wall and posterior portion of inferior turbinate; and the posterior septal branch, which supplies the anterio-inferior face of the sphenoid sinus and posterior septum.
2. Aggressive inferior dissection of the perpendicular plate of the palatine bone during maxillary mega-antrostomy may predispose to significant intraoperative hemorrhage due to its proximity to the posterior lateral nasal branch.
3. Avoid unnecessary or aggressive postoperative debridement of the fresh wound bed or inferior turbinate posterior stump following mega-antrostomy procedures.

Case Presentation

A 23-year-old female with a history of cystic fibrosis presented to the rhinology clinic with a long-standing history of facial pressure and purulent discharge. The patient had undergone endoscopic sinus surgery (ESS) twice previously, most recently 3 years ago. On endoscopic exam, the patient was noted to have thick purulent secretions in the left maxillary sinus that were visualized through the prior antrostomy. CT imaging demonstrated persistent pansinusitis. After counseling about management options, the patient elected to undergo revision ESS with left maxillary mega-antrostomy, for symptomatic benefit in CF-related CRS with

C. J. Massey · V. R. Ramakrishnan (✉)
Department of Otolaryngology, University of Colorado School of Medicine, Aurora, CO, USA
e-mail: Vijay.ramakrishnan@cuanschutz.edu

R. K. Chandra, K. C. Welch (eds.), *Lessons Learned from Rhinologic Procedure Complications*, https://doi.org/10.1007/978-3-030-75323-8_18

chronic purulent drainage [1]. The surgery was uncomplicated, and at the first postoperative appointment 9 days later, the patient was noted to have bothersome obstructive nasal crusting and dry clot emanating from the surgical site, adherent to the posterior inferior turbinate stump (Fig. 18.1). After topical administration of lidocaine and decongestant in the clinic, the clot and crust were removed with minimal effort, and almost immediately the patient began experiencing a large volume bleed from the debrided area. Bleeding slowed with placement of nonabsorbable packing, however, the patient continued to bleed and required placement of two 8-cm polyvinyl acetate packs in the left nasal cavity to achieve temporary hemostasis.

The patient was taken urgently to the OR for control of hemorrhage due to slow continued bleeding despite packing. After intubation and preparation, upon removal of the nasal packs, arterial bleeding was observed from the healing inferior turbinate stump, and this was quickly and successfully controlled with suction cautery. No further bleeding was noted. The patient went on to have an unremarkable postoperative course with eventual improvement in symptoms, and on subsequent follow-up debridement was avoided.

Root Cause Analysis

The bleeding in our case occurred during routine debridement at the first postoperative visit. In a region adjacent to both the sphenopalatine artery and its branches along with the descending palatine artery and its branches, care should be taken prior to removing significant crusts adherent to this anatomical subsite.

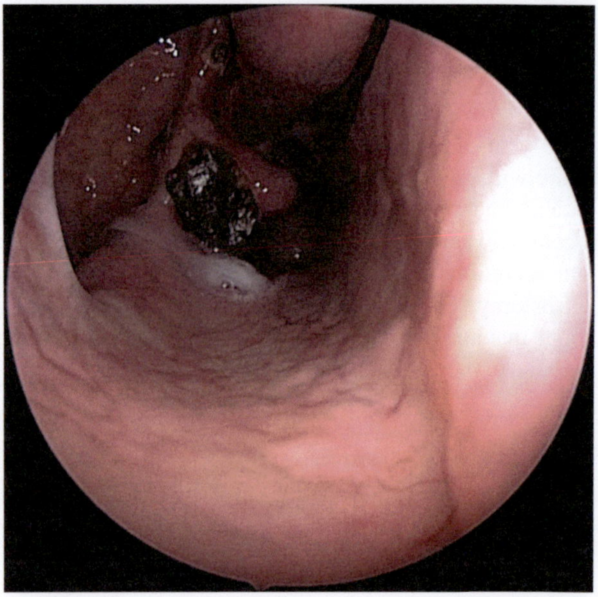

Fig. 18.1 Early postoperative clinic endoscopy after right-sided modified endoscopy medial maxillectomy. The inferior turbinate stump is cauterized during the procedure, and generally displays some degree of scab present in the early postoperative period. This may be adherent to the inferior turbinate branch of the posterior lateral nasal branch of the SPA

Lessons Learned

Maxillary mega-antrostomy, also known as modified endoscopic medial maxillectomy (MEMM), is a procedure that may be indicated for patients with CRS or mucociliary derangement who have recalcitrant maxillary disease despite prior technically proper maxillary antrostomy [2, 3]. In this procedure, the medial wall of the maxillary sinus is removed, along with a portion of the inferior turbinate, so that the sinus opens up on to the floor of nasal cavity. A recent systematic review collecting generally low-quality evidence demonstrated that MEMM is effective in improving symptoms in about 60–80% of cases [4]. A number of the included studies showed a statistically significant improvement in objective outcomes such as CT and endoscopic disease burden. The review deemed that MEMM is generally safe based on an aggregate complication rate of 1.9% (4/211), of which significant postoperative bleeding accounted for 0.5% (1/211).

In this procedure, significant bleeding can occur from resection of the lateral nasal/medial maxillary sinus wall and inferior turbinate due to the rich vascular supply to this region from the sphenopalatine artery (SPA). The SPA stems from the internal maxillary artery, a terminal branch of the external carotid, which passes into the nasal cavity via the sphenopalatine foramen. Although many variations have been reported, it generally gives off two major branches after it enters the nasal cavity: the posterior septal branch, which supplies the face/anterio-inferior wall of the sphenoid sinus and posterior nasal septum; and the posterior lateral nasal branch (PLNB), which supplies the lateral nasal wall and nasal turbinates. It has been estimated that the SPA passes through the sphenopalatine foramen as a single trunk 67–76% of the time [5, 6]; the remainder variants included SPA branching proximal to the foramen, and branching through accessory foramina.

Lee et al. performed a detailed anatomical study of how the lateral nasal wall and turbinates are supplied by the PLNB and how these may impact surgical dissection in this area [7] (Fig. 18.2). For routine maxillary antrostomy, minor arterial bleeding may be encountered with anterior–inferior resection; this area is supplied by the fontanelle subbranch. For MEMM, more significant bleeding may occur as dissection proceeds through the inferior turbinate, which is supplied by a larger inferior turbinate subbranch. Dissection further through the perpendicular plate of the palatine bone carries the greatest risk of massive hemorrhage, as this is where the PLNB generally courses prior to branching. The PLNB can range in diameter from 1.8 to 2.4 mm in this area.

The literature is scant with regard to proper management of SPA bleeding from extended lateral nasal wall resection, such as MEMM, likely due to the infrequency with which this procedure is performed. Most publications discuss management of SPA hemorrhage as it relates to idiopathic epistaxis [8]. In a clinic or emergency room setting where endoscopic visualization and instrumentation is not available or feasible, management of a suspected SPA bleed should be attempted with packing. Longer (8–10 cm) nonabsorbable packs, or Foley catheter balloon packing, are generally needed to reach this area. Frequently, however, bleeding from an SPA source

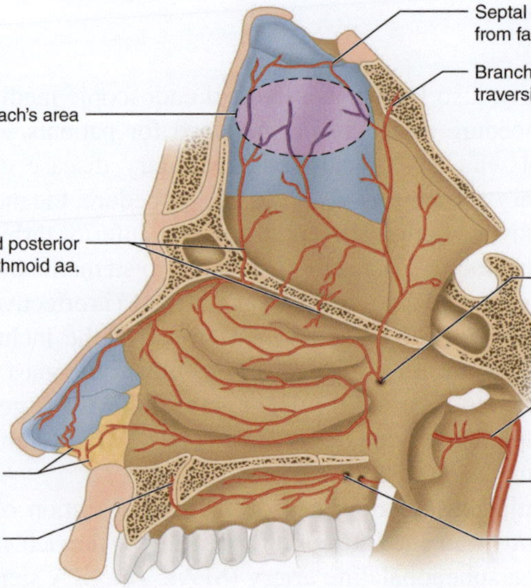

Fig. 18.2 Anatomic distribution of the sphenopalatine artery. Two major branches supply the lateral nasal wall (left) and the septum (right). The lateral nasal wall branch gives significant contribution posteriorly to the turbinates that approximate the surgical field or postoperative crusts that are frequently debrided. Note the course of the posterior septal branch along the arch of the choana below the sphenoid ostium

needs to be controlled in the OR with electrocautery or SPA ligation or in the interventional radiology suite [9].

The bleeding in our case occurred during routine debridement at the first postoperative visit. Postoperative debridement is thought to promote healing and prevent formation of adhesions, although data supporting the practice are limited [10]. Interestingly, while bleeding from postoperative debridement is a known risk of this procedure, a recent Cochrane review compiling data from four studies (152 participants) on this practice did not report any instances of significant bleeding [11]. The authors were not able to conclude whether this finding was due to actual lack of occurrences, or whether the data were just not reported. All studies were of low-quality evidence and carried a high risk of bias.

Awareness of the anatomic location of major SPA branches is critical for the surgeon, as similar occurrences to our case presentation may result from low entry through the middle turbinate basal lamella during total ethmoidectomy or partial middle turbinate resection from the SPA branch to the middle turbinate. Or perhaps more commonly, a large sphenoidotomy that is carried inferiorly may be likely to transect the posterior septal branch. These situations may benefit from focal cautery intraoperatively, or could very well risk postoperative hemorrhage, or hemorrhage with debridement. It is important to note that bipolar coagulation is preferred, or if monopolar suction cautery is required that low setting, focal application, and brief administration time would be ideal to limit energy spread.

Postoperative nasal packing as a preventative measure for bleeding in cases of routine ESS has been studied, but not for MEMM specifically. Routine use of non-absorbable nasal packing or hemostatic agents in ESS has not been shown to be necessary for most cases [12] and may increase patient discomfort postoperatively or potentiate bleeding during packing removal.

Patients who require MEMM for chronic maxillary sinusitis tend to have recalcitrant disease and have often already been managed with multiple rounds of ESS. These patients frequently have altered surgical anatomy, either due to missing landmarks or neo-osteogenesis, which may place them at increased risk for complications. While the complication rate for MEMM seems to be low based on the available evidence, we feel that control and prevention of hemorrhage, both intra- and postoperatively, are important considerations given the high vascularity of the surgical field. The SPA supplies this region with a rich network of branches that directly feeds the inferior turbinate and lateral nasal wall. Aggressive posterio-inferior resection of the inferior turbinate or perpendicular plate of the palatine bone may increase the risk of intraoperative bleeding. Postoperatively, these patients are prone to developing crusts that may lead to adhesion formation if not debrided, much like any other patient undergoing ESS. However, our experience following this case has led us to be much less aggressive in debriding the fresh mega-antrostomy. In fact, postoperative debridement has not been shown to improve quality of life and, apart from bleeding, may cause significant patient discomfort. Secondly, a high-volume bleed from this area in a clinic setting may be hard to control and necessitate urgent OR intervention, placing the patient at high risk for morbidity and creating psychological distress for all persons involved. While all patients undergoing ESS should have thoughtful counseling regarding the risk of bleeding, the risk of a high-volume bleed from MEMM may be higher, and this needs to be emphasized in any surgical consent discussion for this procedure.

References

1. Wang EW, Gullung JL, Schlosser RJ. Modified endoscopic medial maxillectomy for recalcitrant chronic maxillary sinusitis. Int Forum Allergy Rhinol. 2011;1(6):493–7.
2. Woodworth BA, Parker RO, Schlosser RJ. Modified endoscopic medial maxillectomy for chronic maxillary sinusitis. Am J Rhinol. 2006;20(3):317–9.
3. Cho D-Y, Hwang PH. Results of endoscopic maxillary mega-antrostomy in recalcitrant maxillary sinusitis. Am J Rhinol. 2008;22(6):658–62.
4. Loftus CA, Yoo F, Desiato VM, Schlosser RJ, Soler ZM. Treatment of recalcitrant maxillary sinusitis with endoscopic modified medial maxillectomy: a systematic review of safety and efficacy. Am J Rhinol Allergy. 2020;34(1):127–33.
5. Pádua FGM, Voegels RL. Severe posterior epistaxis-endoscopic surgical anatomy. Laryngoscope. 2008;118(1):156–61.
6. Gras-Cabrerizo JR, Ademá-Alcover JM, Gras-Albert JR, Kolanczak K, Montserrat-Gili JR, Mirapeix-Lucas R, et al. Anatomical and surgical study of the sphenopalatine artery branches. Eur Arch Otorhinolaryngol. 2014;271(7):1947–51.

7. Lee HY, Kim H-U, Kim S-S, Son EJ, Kim JW, Cho NH, et al. Surgical anatomy of the sphenopalatine artery in lateral nasal wall. Laryngoscope. 2002;112(10):1813–8.
8. Tunkel DE, Anne S, Payne SC, Ishman SL, Rosenfeld RM, Abramson PJ, et al. Clinical practice guideline: nosebleed (epistaxis). Otolaryngol Head Neck Surg. 2020;162(1_suppl):S1–38.
9. Sireci F, Speciale R, Sorrentino R, Turri-Zanoni M, Nicolotti M, Canevari FR. Nasal packing in sphenopalatine artery bleeding: therapeutic or harmful? Eur Arch Otorhinolaryngol. 2017;274(3):1501–5.
10. Ramakrishnan VR, Suh JD. How necessary are postoperative debridements after endoscopic sinus surgery? Laryngoscope. 2011;121(1):8–9.
11. Tzelnick S, Alkan U, Leshno M, Hwang P, Soudry E. Sinonasal debridement versus no debridement for the postoperative care of patients undergoing endoscopic sinus surgery. Cochrane Database Syst Rev. 2018;11:CD011988.
12. Eliashar R, Gross M, Wohlgelernter J, Sichel J-Y. Packing in endoscopic sinus surgery: is it really required? Otolaryngol Head Neck Surg. 2006;134(2):276–9.

Chapter 19
Bleeding of the Anterior Ethmoid Artery

Amarbir S. Gill, Toby O. Steele, and Jeremiah A. Alt

Clinical Pearls

1. Utilize known radiologic landmarks such as the supraorbital cell and the Keros classification to identify the anterior ethmoid artery (AEA) on preoperative imaging.
2. Adhere to good functional endoscopic sinus surgery (FESS) principles of maintaining a "dry" surgical field to optimize visualization.
3. Prepare to execute a standardized and stepwise approach to management of intraoperative transection of the AEA.

Case Presentation

A 62-year-old woman with a history of chronic rhinosinusitis (CRS) with nasal polyposis (CRSwNP) and a prior surgical history of bilateral complete functional endoscopic sinus surgery (FESS), presented with persistent CRS-related symptoms. After failing appropriate medical management the patient elected revision FESS. The patient was taken to the operating room for an elective revision bilateral FESS with septoplasty. The surgeon began by performing a routine septoplasty followed by an uneventful complete FESS on the left side. On the contralateral side,

A. S. Gill · T. O. Steele
Department of Otolaryngology – Head and Neck Surgery, University of California, Davis, Sacramento, CA, USA

J. A. Alt (✉)
Division of Otolaryngology – Head and Neck Surgery, Rhinology-Sinus and Skull Base Surgery Program, Department of Surgery, University of Utah School of Medicine, Salt Lake City, UT, USA
e-mail: jeremial.alt@hsc.utah.edu

R. K. Chandra, K. C. Welch (eds.), *Lessons Learned from Rhinologic Procedure Complications*, https://doi.org/10.1007/978-3-030-75323-8_19

the surgeon encountered a moderate amount of venous oozing due to the significant polyp burden and osteitis, which substantially reduced visualization. The surgeon utilized the microdebrider during his posterior to anterior dissection along the skull base to remove polyps, as well as residual ethmoid lamella. While working along the anterior ethmoid skull base immediately posterior to the frontal sinus, the surgeon noticed a sudden increase in pulsatile bleeding. This required packing the nose and sinus cavities with pledgets soaked in 1:1000 epinephrine in an attempt to control the bleeding. The surgeon, acknowledging the proximity to the orbit and the anterior ethmoid artery (AEA), correctly evaluated the right eye, which demonstrated a rapidly progressing proptosis and tense globe compared to the left eye. The AEA had been inadvertently transected and retracted into the right orbit resulting in ongoing intraorbital hemorrhage. Given signs of orbital compartment syndrome, the surgeon proceeded with a canthotomy and cantholysis, which reversed the proptosis and eye firmness, after which the case was terminated. The patient was awakened and was found to have suffered no vision complications.

Root Cause Analysis

Prevalence

The overall risk of major complications from FESS is noted to be approximately 3% [1]. Stankiewicz et al. noted the risk of an orbital hematoma to be 0.06% across 3402 cases over 25 years [1]. The authors reported that revision surgery, extensive disease, and nasal polyposis increased the likelihood of a complication [1]. Krings et al. subsequently performed a large database analysis of 78,944 patients and demonstrated an overall complication rate of 0.36% and an orbital complication rate of 0.23%, with no significant difference between primary and revision surgeries [2].

It is possible that during FESS in patients with significant inflammatory burden (i.e., polyp load, bony osteitis), surgical field visualization may be impaired from heavy bleeding leading to the increased potential for iatrogenic injury. It is imperative that the endoscopic sinus surgeon anticipate and preempt the potential for orbital, skull base, and vessel injury in this situation.

Prevention

Several critical principles of FESS can assist in maintaining a field that is as bloodless as possible in these challenging cases. First, a reverse Trendelenberg position has been shown to reduce bleeding after 2 h as compared to controls [3]. Second, visualization of the surgical field has been shown to improve with the use of both preoperative oral prednisone, and total intravenous anesthesia (TIVA) with propofol, which can be supplemented with a remifentanil infusion. The latter provides controlled hypotension in these cases [3, 4]. There is also interest in the use of dexmedetomidine as an alternative to remifentanil. Ongoing research suggests similar effects on blood loss, with potentially superior pain control in the immediate postoperative setting [4, 5]. Third, maintaining good "sink control" is important in FESS, which means regularly suctioning blood from the ethmoid, sphenoid, and maxillary sinuses and nasopharynx. This provides a "sink" for fresh blood to drain so that it does not obscure the surgeon's field. Finally, topical 1:1000 epinephrine has been shown to be an excellent vasoconstrictor, and superior to oxymetazoline. It is generally considered safe to use, with caution advised in patients with known history of cardiac comorbidities [6, 7].

Role of Preoperative Imaging

Diligent study of preoperative imaging is absolutely critical to anticipate potential complex anatomy or anatomic variants, which can pay dividends in avoiding inadvertent intraoperative AEA injury. Error et al. analyzed the implementation of a standardized preoperative radiologic checklist to critically evaluate sinus anatomy. The authors demonstrated a significant improvement in recognition of sinus anatomy variations among otolaryngology residents; accuracy increased from 24% to 84% ($p < 0.001$) in this single-blinded cohort study [8]. Although the AEA is commonly located within the skull base adjacent to the superior oblique muscle [9], studies have demonstrated that in up to 40% of patients the AEA will lie below the skull base, often within its mesentery or with frank dehiscence [9]. When present, the AEA has been described to form the "nipple sign" within its bony mesentery, located at the junction between the superior orbit and skull base (see Fig. 19.1).

Radiologic Landmarks for AEA

The following major landmarks are associated with a low-lying AEA and should be assessed routinely in preoperative imaging: presence of a supraorbital ethmoid cell (SOEC), anterior posterior diameter from the anterior wall of the frontal sinus to the skull base (AFP), and the Keros classification [10]. In the presence of an SOEC, the AEA will be below the skull base in 53.8% of cases [11]; in these cases, the exact location of the AEA will be posterior to the SOEC [11]. Conversely, when the SOEC is not present, the AEA is below the skull base in only 18% of cases. [11] Data have demonstrated that up to 56% of patients can have supraorbital pneumatization [12]. Finally, Poteet et al. demonstrated that a Keros 3 classification, compared to a Keros 1 and 2, was significantly more likely to be associated with an AEA below the skull base [13]. Recognizing these critical landmarks on preoperative imaging and intraoperatively can help avoid injury. In the described case, preoperative CT scan

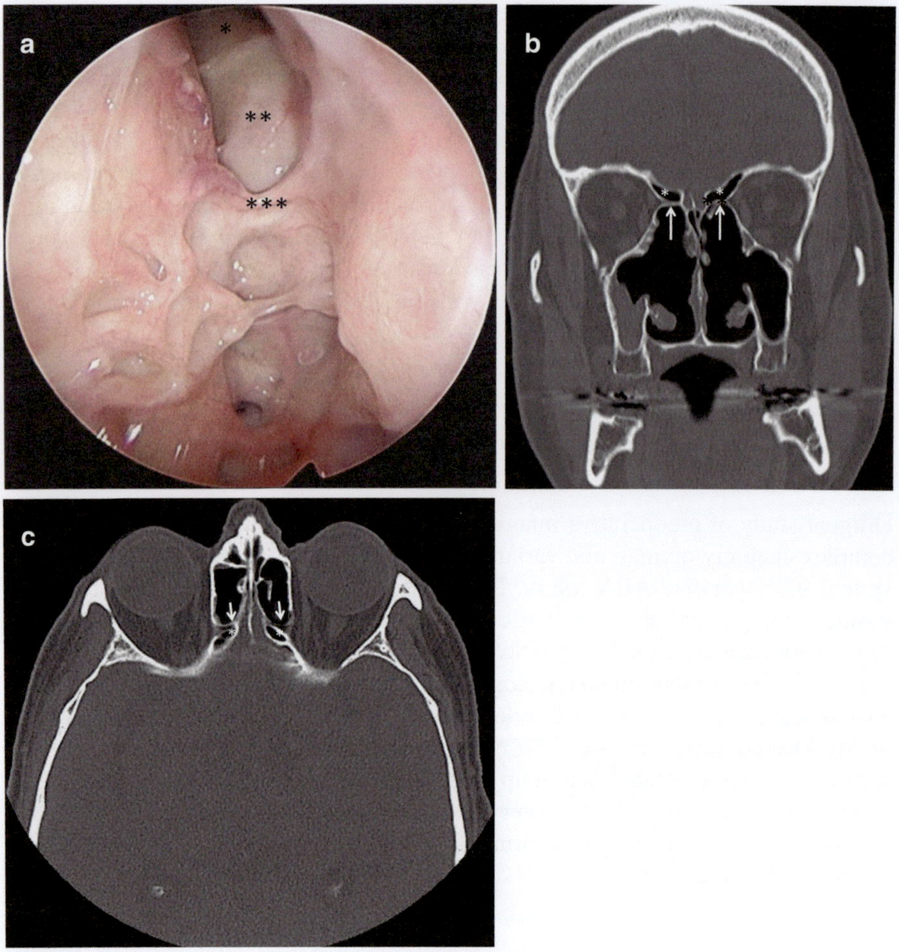

Fig. 19.1 (**a**) Endoscopic demonstration of the anterior ethmoid artery (AEA) suspended within its mesentery, and its relationship to the supraorbital ethmoid cell (SOEC) and frontal sinus (FS) along the skull base. Legend: *FS, **SOEC, ***AEA. (**b**) Corresponding computed tomography (CT) in coronal orientation demonstrating bilateral supraorbital ethmoid cells (SOEC) (asterisk), and bilateral "nipple sign" (white arrows). The latter radiologic findings highlight the anterior ethmoid artery (AEA), which is suspended within its mesentery and thus at higher risk of iatrogenic injury. (**c**) Corresponding computed tomography (CT) in axial orientation demonstrating the relationship between the anterior ethmoid artery (AEA) (white arrows) and the supraorbital ethmoid cell (SOEC) (asterisk), when present

demonstrated that the anterior ethmoid artery was within the skull base on the left, but suspended from the skull base within its mesentery on the right with an associated SOEC.

Lessons Learned

The surgeon must be prepared to execute a standardized and stepwise approach to management of intraoperative transection of the AEA. These include recognition, localization, cautery, and various means to decompress the orbit. However, when it has become clear that the AEA has retracted into the orbital cone with the development of compartment syndrome, decompression becomes the priority, which is first accomplished via lateral canthotomy and cantholysis.

Recognition and Localization

First and foremost, recognition of the injury and its severity are critical. Signs may range from sudden, potentially pulsatile bleeding when working along the ethmoid skull base, to those of orbital compartment syndrome, where an actively hemorrhaging AEA retracts into the orbit. When AEA injury is suspected from bleeding in the surgical field, a 70° or 90° curved suction can be used to pinpoint the exact location, noting that the location of the AEA is generally posterior to the posterior table of the frontal sinus along the anterior ethmoid skull base [14].

However, if orbital signs are observed, the surgeon must be aware that this can become an ophthalmologic emergency within minutes. The affected eye may demonstrate proptosis/firmness and become "rock hard"; ecchymosis, chemosis and a dilated pupil might be observed [1].

Treatment Algorithm

AEA hemorrhage can be addressed in a stepwise fashion, starting with the most conservative intervention and quickly graduating to more invasive means for control, if necessary (see Fig. 19.2 for a suggested algorithm).

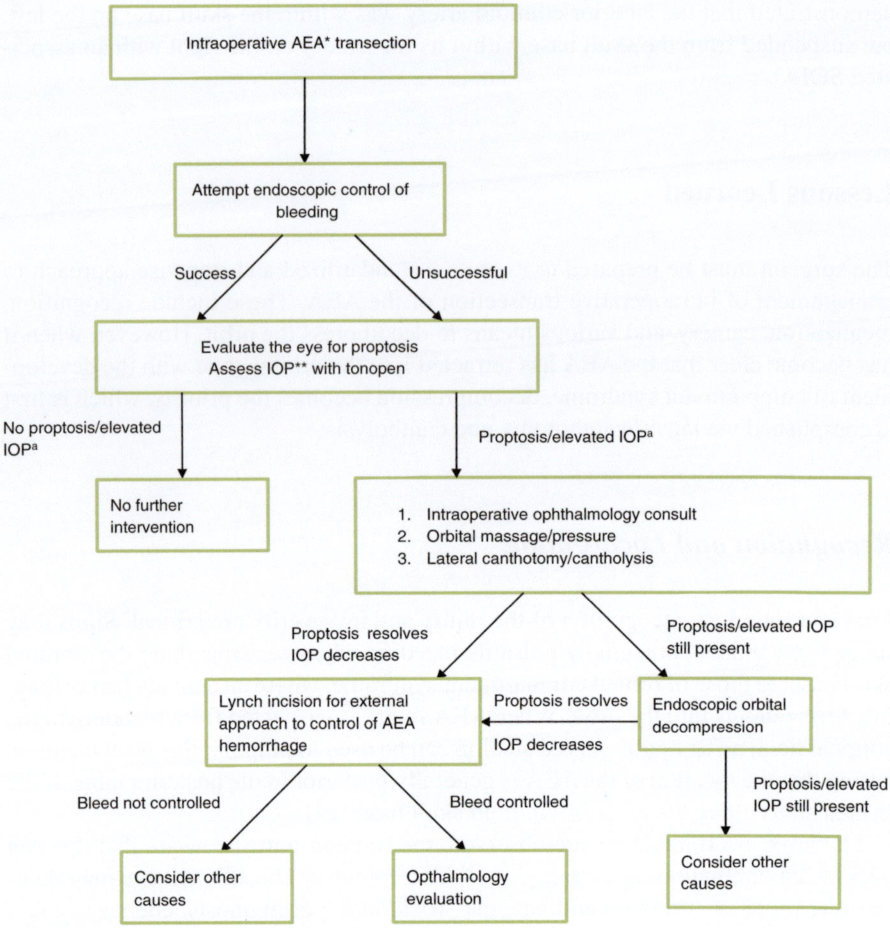

Fig. 19.2 Management of iatrogenic injury to the anterior ethmoid artery: a stepwise algorithm. Legend: AEA – anterior ethmoid artery, IOP – intraocular pressure. [a]Elevated IOP necessitating intervention: >40 mmHg

Bipolar Versus Monopolar Cautery

In the described case, the surgeon immediately recognized injury to the AEA and attempted to control the bleeding with bipolar cautery. However, this was not successful, as the AEA had retracted into the orbit. This situation is more likely to occur if the artery was transected bluntly and closer to the orbit as opposed to the cribiform [9]. The surgeon then attempted to control the bleeding with monopolar suction bovie; it is critical to keep in mind that use of the suction bovie has the theoretical risk of creating an iatrogenic CSF leak along the skull base given the high-energy transfer to surrounding tissue, such as the eye, dura, and brain. Furthermore, one must be aware that the superior oblique muscle abuts the AEA as it exits from the orbit; it could theoretically be injured with aggressive cauterization in this area [1, 15].

When Cautery Fails – Managing the Orbit?

When the AEA has already retracted into the orbit, the aforementioned techniques at endoscopic cautery typically fail to control the bleeding and within minutes the eye becomes proptotic.

Stankiewicz et al. advocate for orbital massage as the first step when orbital hematoma is suspected [1, 16]. In their series of 3402 cases, the group reported 20 total orbital hematomas with only three associated with AEA injury. Orbital massage was the primary initial treatment and successfully managed the bleed alongside endoscopic control of the hemorrhage in one out of three cases of AEA injury [1]. Ultimately, the other two cases required additional surgical intervention with canthotomy/cantholysis or orbital decompression, due to lack of improvement in eye firmness. Although two out of three patients were noted to have temporary vision loss, none had long-term vision loss. The authors argue that there is a limited role for medical management in a suspected *arterial* orbital hematoma, as the onset of action for intraocular pressure (IOP)-reducing medications such as timolol drops, acetazolamide, and mannitol is 20–30 min.

Role of the Lateral Canthotomy/Cantholysis

It is important to remember that a lateral canthotomy with cantholysis is advocated when IOP is greater than 40 mmHg [15, 17]. Although in monkeys, retina ischemia time has been shown to be around 90 min [18], it is theorized that in an arterial hematoma, as opposed to a venous bleed, the time period for irreversible vision loss may be much less, around 15–30 min [1]. An emergent ophthalmology consult in the operating room (OR) may not be available; thus, every endoscopic sinus surgeon should be comfortable making the decision to perform this procedure (see Fig. 19.3 for an illustration of the procedure) [15, 17]. It is also important to note that although immediate measurement of intraocular pressures in the OR is ideal, this may not be available, and the decision to proceed with canthotomy/cantholysis may be predicated on progressive firmness of the eye despite initial pressure/massage.

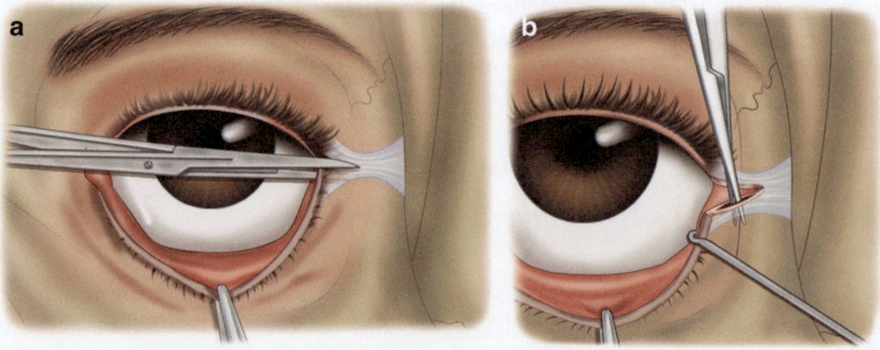

Fig. 19.3 (**a**) Medical illustration of a lateral canthotomy. The skin over the lateral canthus is cut with scissors. (**b**) Medical illustration of a lateral cantholysis. Once the skin overlying the lateral canthus is cut, the attachment of the lateral canthal tendon onto the lateral orbital rim can be palpated via "bowstring" of the tendon. Scissors are then turned vertically and used to cut this tendon from its attachment, thus increasing the laxity of the inferior eyelid and effectively decreasing intraocular pressures

Endoscopic Orbital Decompression

If canthotomy/cantholysis fails to control the elevated IOP or resolve the proptosis and firmness, the surgeon may consider endoscopic orbital decompression of the lamina with incision of the periorbita to decrease the pressure on the globe, given impending vision loss [1, 19].

Moreover, by taking down the lamina in this fashion, one may be able to identify the retracted AEA stump between the periorbita and the lamina. Once identified, the stump can be bipolared for easy control of hemorrhage. If the stump is not seen here, it may have further retracted into the orbit itself, necessitating an external approach [19].

External Approach to the AEA for Control of Hemorrhage

Once the AEA has retracted into the periorbita, control may be established in a stepwise fashion, starting with endoscopic orbital decompression and graduating to an external approach [1, 17]. In the described case, having temporarily reversed the proptosis with the canthotomy/cantholysis, but unable to identify the AEA stump even after orbital decompression, the surgeon proceeded to an external approach to control the AEA. This can be achieved by first designing a 1 cm curvilinear incision centered between the nasal dorsum and medial canthus. The goal is to position the incision over the frontoethmoidal suture line, as this will help approximate the location of the AEA. The incision is injected with 1% lidocaine with 1:100,000 epinephrine. A 15-blade is used to incise skin and subcutaneous tissue, taking care to clip the angular artery/vein as dissection is carried deeper. Inferiorly, the limit of dissection is the lacrimal sac. The frontoethmoidal suture line is identified along the superior aspect of the lacrimal bone. The periosteum is incised and with the help of a 0° endoscope, the suture line is followed posteriorly using a Cottle or Freer elevator until the AEA is identified, at which point it is controlled with two hemoclips or bipolar cautery [20].

Medial orbital wall decompression can also be approached externally via a transcuruncular approach. The caruncle is retracted medially and the incision site is injected with 1% lidocaine with 1:100,000 epinephrine. A 15-blade is used to incise the conjunctiva. Small curved scissors are then used to bluntly dissect down onto the posterior lacrimal crest; the medial orbital wall is located just posterior to this bony prominence and, once identified, it can easily be exposed to facilitate bony removal and subsequent periorbital incision for decompression. Care must be taken not to carry the dissection further posterior to the medial orbital wall, as this can result in injury to the medial rectus muscle, which attaches to the periorbita here. Since the AEA transverses the periorbita in this same region, the transcaruncular incision can also be used to identify and control hemorrhage from the AEA at the same time [21].

References

1. Stankiewicz JA, Lal D, Connor M, Welch K. Complications in endoscopic sinus surgery for chronic rhinosinusitis: a 25-year experience. Laryngoscope. 2011;121:2684–701.
2. Krings JG, Kallogjeri D, Wineland A, Nepple KG, Piccirillo JF, Getz AE. Complications of primary and revision functional endoscopic sinus surgery for chronic rhinosinusitis. Laryngoscope. 2014;124:838–45.
3. Rodriguez Valiente A, Roldan Fidalgo A, Laguna Ortega D. Bleeding control in endoscopic sinus surgery: a systematic review of the literature. Rhinology. 2013;51:298–305.
4. Amorocho MC, Fat I. Anesthetic techniques in endoscopic sinus and skull base surgery. Otolaryngol Clin N Am. 2016;49:531–47.
5. Lee HS, Yoon HY, Jin HJ, Hwang SH. Can dexmedetomidine influence recovery profiles from general anesthesia in nasal surgery? Otolaryngol Head Neck Surg. 2018;158:43–53.
6. Orlandi RR, Warrier S, Sato S, Han JK. Concentrated topical epinephrine is safe in endoscopic sinus surgery. Am J Rhinol Allergy. 2010;24:140–2.
7. Kuan EC, Tajudeen BA, Bhandarkar ND, St John MA, Palmer JN, Adappa ND. Is topical epinephrine safe for hemostasis in endoscopic sinus surgery? Laryngoscope. 2019;129:1–3.
8. Error M, Ashby S, Orlandi RR, Alt JA. Single-blinded prospective implementation of a preoperative imaging checklist for endoscopic sinus surgery. Otolaryngol Head Neck Surg. 2018;158:177–80.
9. Eloy JA, Svider PF, Setzen M. Clinical pearls in endoscopic sinus surgery: key steps in preventing and dealing with complications. Am J Otolaryngol. 2014;35:324–8.
10. Sjogren PP, Waghela R, Ashby S, Wiggins RH, Orlandi RR, Alt JA. International frontal sinus anatomy classification and anatomic predictors of low-lying anterior ethmoidal arteries. Am J Rhinol Allergy. 2017;31:174–6.
11. Li M, Sharbel DD, White B, Tadros SY, Kountakis SE. Reliability of the supraorbital ethmoid cell vs Keros classification in predicting the course of the anterior ethmoid artery. Int Forum Allergy Rhinol. 2019;9:821–4.

12. Abdullah B, Lim EH, Husain S, Snidvongs K, Wang Y. Anatomical variations of anterior ethmoidal artery and their significance in endoscopic sinus surgery: a systematic review. Surg Radiol Anat. 2019;41:491–9.
13. Poteet PS, Cox MD, Wang RA, Fitzgerald RT, Kanaan A. Analysis of the relationship between the location of the anterior ethmoid artery and Keros classification. Otolaryngol Head Neck Surg. 2017;157:320–4.
14. Jang DW, Lachanas VA, White LC, Kountakis SE. Supraorbital ethmoid cell: a consistent landmark for endoscopic identification of the anterior ethmoidal artery. Otolaryngol Head Neck Surg. 2014;151:1073–7.
15. Dallan I, Tschabitscher M, Castelnuovo P, et al. Management of severely bleeding ethmoidal arteries. J Craniofac Surg. 2009;20:450–4.
16. Stankiewicz JA, Chow JM. Two faces of orbital hematoma in intranasal (endoscopic) sinus surgery. Otolaryngol Head Neck Surg. 1999;120:841–7.
17. Graham SM, Nerad JA. Orbital complications in endoscopic sinus surgery using powered instrumentation. Laryngoscope. 2003;113:874–8.
18. Hayreh SS, Kolder HE, Weingeist TA. Central retinal artery occlusion and retinal tolerance time. Ophthalmology. 1980;87:75–8.
19. Snyderman C, Carrau RL. Bleeding during endoscopic sinus surgery. In: Meyers EN, editor. Operative otolaryngology: head and neck surgery. Edinburgh: Saunders Elsevier; 2008.
20. Snyderman C, Carrau RL. Epistaxis. In: Myers EN, editor. Operative otolaryngology: head and neck surgery. Edinburgh: Saunders Elsevier; 2008.
21. Graham SM, Thomas RD, Carter KD, Nerad JA. The transcaruncular approach to the medial orbital wall. Laryngoscope. 2002;112:986–9.

Chapter 20
Carotid Artery Injury During Skull Base Surgery

Mathew N. Geltzeiler and Eric W. Wang

Clinical Pearls

1. Management of a carotid injury during skull base surgery requires an experienced team that can work together efficiently.
2. Preoperative assessment of vascular anatomy, tumor involvement and cerebral perfusion, plus intraoperative image guidance and neurophysiologic monitoring can all help with decision making.
3. Intraoperative hemostasis must be followed by additional evaluation and management in the neurointerventional radiology suite.

Case Presentation

A 48-year-old female presents with diplopia and a partial right oculomotor nerve palsy. Magnetic resonance imaging (MRI) revealed an enhancing, dural-based lesion in the central skull base consistent with a meningioma. The lesion shows involvement of the bilateral cavernous sinuses and internal carotid arteries with the majority of the tumor bulk and vessel encasement on the right (Fig. 20.1). The patient was taken to the operating room for an endoscopic endonasal approach to the sella and middle cranial fossa. Wide exposure to access the tumor was achieved without difficulty. During tumor dissection in the right cavernous sinus, a small laceration of the right internal carotid artery occurred (Fig. 20.2a). The entire operating room team was notified. Hemostasis was initially controlled with direct pressure utilizing cottonoids. The anesthesiology team maintained normotension with

M. N. Geltzeiler · E. W. Wang (✉)
University of Pittsburgh Medical Center, The Eye & Ear Institute,
Pittsburgh, PA, USA
e-mail: wangew@upmc.edu

R. K. Chandra, K. C. Welch (eds.), *Lessons Learned from Rhinologic Procedure Complications*, https://doi.org/10.1007/978-3-030-75323-8_20

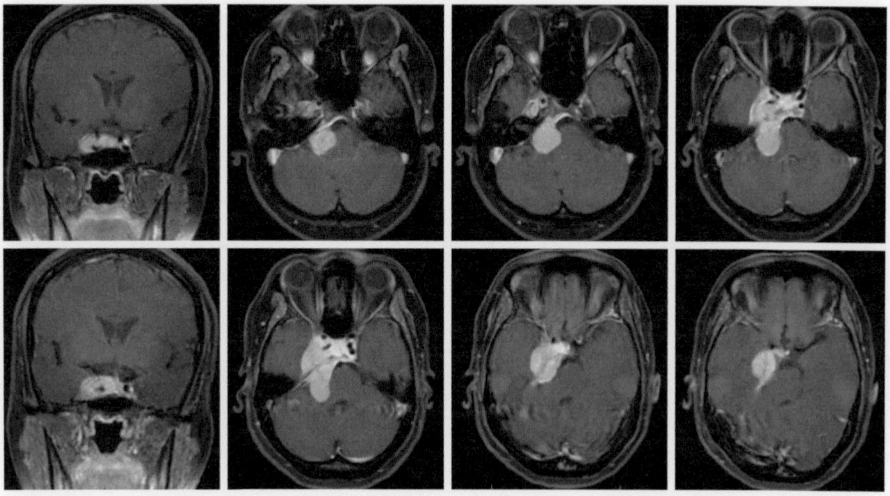

Fig. 20.1 Coronal and axial T1 MRI with gadolinium enhancement of a right-sided sphenocavernous meningioma with involvement of the bilateral cavernous sinuses. The meningioma encases the right cavernous internal carotid artery and abuts the left cavernous segment of the left internal carotid artery. Both the tumor involvement and location of the meningioma create a high-risk scenario for internal carotid artery injury

fluid resuscitation and iatrogenic support. Blood products including packed RBC, platelets, and fresh frozen plasma were made immediately available. The carotid artery was reconstructed with an aneurysm clip via a single shaft clip applier (Fig. 20.2b). The patency of the vessel was confirmed with micro-Doppler both proximally and distally (Fig. 20.2b). Somatosensory evoked potentials (SSEPs) remained unchanged. The tumor dissection was aborted and the clip was covered with an abdominal fat graft (Fig. 20.2c). The reconstruction was completed with a nasoseptal flap (Fig. 20.2d). Standard reconstruction including surgicel, gelfoam, and Merocel sponges were used. The intubated patient was taken to the neurointerventional radiology (neuroIR) suite. The initial angiogram revealed a stenotic yet patient cavernous carotid artery (Fig. 20.3a). This was felt to be secondary to thrombus formation, so the patient was therapeutically anticoagulated with heparin. Four days later, repeat angiogram showed improved vascular patency (Fig. 20.3b). The patient recovered well without any cerebral ischemic event or iatrogenic cranial neuropathy.

Root Cause Analysis

There are several learning points form this case. Injury to the internal carotid artery (ICA) was anticipated in this case as the tumor involved the ICA bilaterally and circumferentially encased the vessel on the right. A preoperative balloon test occlusion (BTO) was performed and passed bilaterally. The team was prepared for

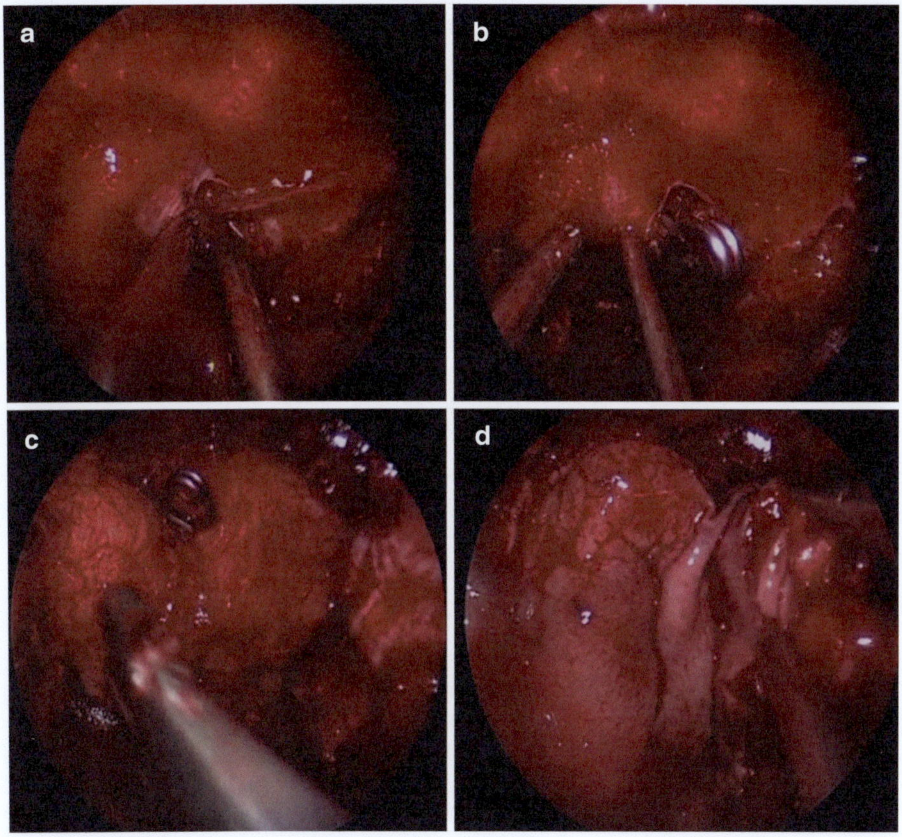

Fig. 20.2 (**a**) Intraoperative endoscopic view of the small laceration of the right internal carotid artery in the cavernous segment. Note the use of suction devices to direct the blood flow away from the endoscope to maintain visualization. (**b**) Reconstruction of the right internal carotid artery with an aneurysm clip. This was placed with a single shaft clip applier after achieving proximal arterial control. Vessel patency was established using a micro-Doppler ultrasound. (**c**) Reconstruction of the skull base defect must take into account the projection of the aneurysm clip. Abdominal fat is used to fill the space surrounding the aneurysm clip to prevent tenting of the vascularized nasoseptal flap. (**d**) Final endoscopic view of nasoseptal flap coverage of the skull base defect and aneurysm clip

possible vascular injury by having a preoperative discussion amongst the operating surgeons, anesthesiologist, nurses, surgical technicians, and neurophysiologist. Large-gauge vascular access was obtained prior to the case and an arterial line was inserted to monitor hemodynamics. Blood products were available. SSEPs were continuously monitored and image guidance was used. During dissection, wide exposure was achieved and bimanual microdissection with dynamic endoscopy was employed. The micro-Doppler and aneurysm clips were available in the room. This preparation allowed for a coordinated and controlled response to an inherently stressful and challenging situation.

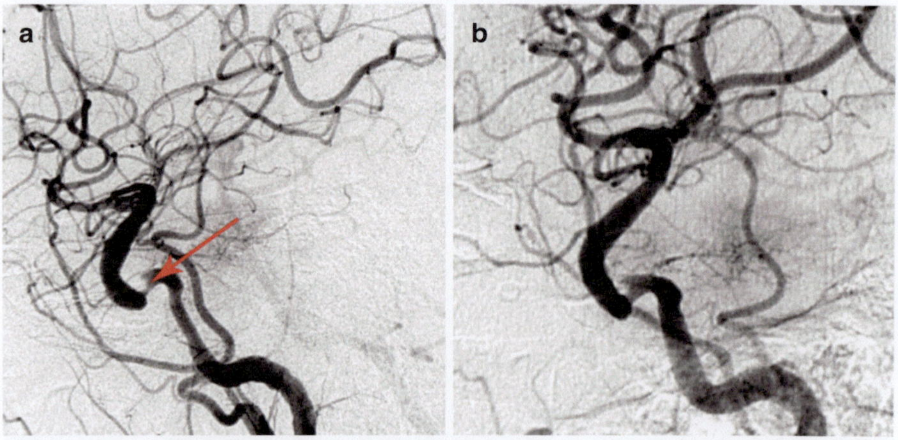

Fig. 20.3 (**a**) Immediate postoperative angiogram after repair of the internal carotid artery injury with an aneurysm clip demonstrates a narrowed yet patent cavernous internal carotid artery. (**b**) After treatment with heparin anticoagulation for 4 days, a repeat angiogram demonstrates improved vascular patency as thrombus from the arterial manipulation has resolved

Hemostasis was initially achieved with cottonoid packing but was transitioned to an aneurysm clip. Direct packing of the injured vessel with crushed muscle is an excellent alternative. Vascular patency was confirmed with micro-Doppler but the adverse event required a formal angiogram in the neurointerventional suite. Prior to leaving the OR, however, dural reconstruction was achieved by protecting the aneurysm clip with an abdominal fat graft and overlaying a nasoseptal flap. Once in the neuro-IR suite, vessel patency was confirmed by the vessel appeared stenotic. The stenosis was felt secondary to thrombus and because there were no SSEP changes, the patient was therapeutically anticoagulated. After day 4, the vessel patency improved allowing for salvage of this vessel.

Lessons Learned

Endoscopic sinus surgery is a safe and efficacious treatment modality for various diseases of the paranasal sinuses. Over the past two decades, advances in endoscopic techniques have grown to include expanded procedures of the skull base. As the type and complexity of cases have grown, vascular management has become an increasingly important component to surgical planning and operative techniques. The internal carotid artery, in particular, is a prominent surgical landmark and within the operative field during the vast majority of sphenoid sinus and skull base surgeries. While the risk of carotid injury is extremely low during sinus surgery, the risks during pituitary surgery and expanded skull base procedure are approximately 1% and 5–9%, respectively [1, 2]. The consequences of vascular injury during skull base surgery can be devastating. The purpose of this chapter is to discuss the

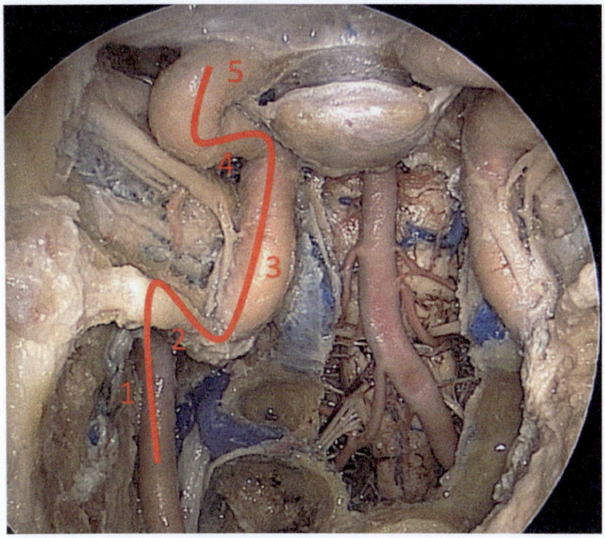

Fig. 20.4 Cadaveric dissection with endoscopic visualization of the course of the internal carotid artery. Note the genus of the internal carotid artery. Starting proximally in the parapharyngeal carotid artery, the vessel then enters the petrous bone in the petrous segment of the carotid artery. At the foramen lacerum, the vessel turns superiorly in the 3rd paraclival segment, labeled 3. This is a higher risk area of injury given the vessel exposure in the transclival approaches. The carotid then enters the cavernous sinus where it is protected by the venous sinus itself except when tumor involves the cavernous sinus itself. Finally, the carotid again becomes more superficial in the 5th segment referred to as the parasellar segment. For sellar and pituitary surgery, this is the segment at high risk of injury

strategies to both prevent and manage internal carotid artery injuries during endoscopic endonasal procedures.

The primary strategy to managing vascular injury is to first prevent it. Prevention begins with a working knowledge of anatomical course of the carotid artery within the skull base. The internal carotid artery can be divided into five segments. The vessel begins extracranially as the parapharyngeal segment enters the skull laterally at the carotid canal and quickly turns anteromedial (Fig. 20.4, #1). The vessel next runs horizontally within the petrous temporal bone (horizontal or petrous segment) (Fig. 20.4, #2). The carotid then turns superiorly at foramen lacerum and runs vertically within the clivus (paraclival segment) (Fig. 20.4, #3) and then is surrounded within the cavernous sinus (cavernous segment or parasellar segment) (Fig. 20.4, #4). Lastly, the carotid becomes intradural (supraclinoidal segment) before anastomosing with the ophthalmic artery and Circle of Willis (Fig. 20.4, #5). Understanding this anatomy is critical for all surgical team members.

The most commonly injured sites are the parasellar carotid and the lacerum segment [3]. The parasellar carotid is routinely encountered during pituitary surgery. Drilling the sphenoid bone off the sella, cavernous sinus and carotid itself should be done with caution as the carotid siphon places the vessel at its most anterior at this segment. Additionally, the bone overlying the carotid prominence may be dehiscent. The vidian nerve can be used as a useful landmark for foramen lacerum [4]. The nerve runs in the pterygoid canal before passing superiolateral to the second genu of the carotid artery. When performing any dissection in the coronal plane via a transpterygoid approach that requires drilling of the lacerum segment, intimate knowledge of the relationships between the lacerum segment of the carotid, the vidian canal, foramen rotundum, the petrosphenoidal fissure, and the lingual process of the sphenoid bone is essential. Lastly, during sellar and suprasellar exposures, the superior and inferior hypophyseal arteries (small branches off the supraclinoidal and cavernous segments, respectively) can be injured or avulsed from the main vessel which can result in a sidewall injury.

Careful examination of vascular anatomy on preoperative imaging is crucial for safely performing surgery. For inflammatory sinonasal surgery, a computed tomography (CT) scan without contrast is typically ordered while for skull base surgery, a CT angiogram can provide a more detailed examination of the course of the carotid artery. Magnetic resonance (MR) images and MR angiography can also be obtained. When examining these images, the course of the carotid artery should be evaluated. Any bony dehiscence over the carotid artery should be noted. While dehiscence can be commonly seen, underlying carotid pseudoaneurysms can also be present. During neoplastic surgery, the tumor may be in close proximity or encase the carotid artery and other intracranial vessels. The tumor may also displace these vessels from their typical course. When planning a surgical approach, understanding how to achieve broad exposure is critical for performing microsurgical dissection and achieving adequate vascular control. If extensive dissection on the carotid artery is planned, a preoperative balloon test occlusion (BTO) should be considered to evaluate contralateral cerebral profusion. Data gathered from the BTO can be used to assess the risk of cerebral ischemic events in the event of carotid sacrifice. If a patient fails BTO, the surgical team may consider altering the goals of surgery or performing a preoperative bypass [3]. Given that BTO is associated with a small risk of morbidity, this test is usually reserved for high-risk patients (i.e., malignancies, recurrent or previously radiated tumors that are adjacent to the carotid). During surgery, image-guidance systems can be utilized to identify vascular anatomy. A micro-Doppler can also be employed. Discussions about the imaging finding among the surgical team prior to the operation allows for an incisive and cohesive operative plan.

Vascular injury may occur during sinus surgery or expanded skull base procedures. Injury during sinus surgery presents a fundamentally different set of challenges than during a skull base procedure as the case may be performed in the outpatient setting with different resources available. Additionally, sinus surgery is typically performed by a single surgeon, so the ability to manage severe bleeding while maintaining adequate visualization is limited. Preoperatively, the surgeon should examine the sphenoid bone to assess for abnormalities in the carotid vasculature including dehiscence of the overlying sphenoid bone or pseudoaneurysm. Image-guidance systems can be particularly useful if anatomic abnormalities are noted. During sphenoidotomy, care should be taken to avoid blind instrumentation within the sinus. If a vascular injury does occur, directly packing the injured area usually with cottonoids is critical to achieve hemostasis. As mentioned, visualization may be challenging. While an attempt to gain temporary hemostasis is underway, anesthesia should ensure adequate intravenous access is achieved and resuscitation has begun. Maintaining adequate blood pressure is also critical for intracranial perfusion. Additional blood products should be ordered. Once the hemorrhage is controlled, the next priority is an immediate angiogram in the interventional neuroradiology suite. There, the interventionalist can evaluate the extent of injury and provide numerous options for vascular control including stenting and vascular sacrifice.

Skull base surgical cases involve a team of otolaryngology and neurosurgery that presents its own unique opportunities and challenges. Intimate knowledge of the anatomy by all operative surgeons is critical for success. Risk of injury can occur during all phases of endoscopic skull base surgery including approach, tumor dissection, and possibly even reconstruction. During the surgical approach, bone removal with a high-speed drill can often necessitate removing the bone of the medial clinoid, carotid canal, and cavernous sinus. Drilling bone by the carotid and cavernous sinus should be done with a diamond drill rather than a cutting burr. Similarly, the risk of internal carotid injury is present during tumor dissection. Preoperative evaluation of the relationship between the tumor and the internal carotid artery in all segments is critical. Encasement of any vessel is important to recognize preoperatively and is an added risk factor. Tumor dissection should also be undertaken with great care intracranially. Whether performing internal debulking or extracapsular tumor dissection, bimanual microdissection technique remains paramount. Dissection of intracranial vasculature and cranial nerves requires bimanual, microscopic dissection techniques, which can only be achieved by effective communication and teamwork. Dynamic endoscopy is critically important to maintaining visualization. More experienced teams can function with a speed and efficiency that directly translates to the necessary skills in managing a vascular accident.

Skull bases cases are performed in the inpatient setting where resources of higher acuity are available. In cases with a higher likelihood of vascular injury, venous access, arterial lines, neurophysiologic monitoring, Doppler ultrasounds, and image guidance should all be routinely employed. If a case has a particularly high risk of vascular injury, a preoperative balloon test occlusion (BTO) should be performed. Blood productions should be available as should ready communication with the neuro-interventional radiology team. Some centers prefer to have vascular clamps (aneurysm clips) available in the operating room to achieve proximally and distal vascular control. Other teams choose to utilize direct vascular pressure with pledgets and/or crushed muscle as their method of temporary control prior to intravascular intervention. Regardless of the chosen modality, an a priori plan should be in place and well understood by all team members including the surgeons, anesthesiologist, scrub technicians, and circulating nurses. Effective planning and communication during these times greatly facilitate speed and efficiency.

Injury to the carotid artery itself results in profound bleeding making visualization and instrumentation challenging. The blood loss is rapid and the risk of hypovolemia is present. The field of view may only be visible momentarily making surgical proficiency and teamwork paramount. A cotton patty should be used initially to tamponade the initial injury until a more definitive approach is applied to reduce blood loss. During these events, the team must carefully weigh the risks of decreasing vascular flow to aid with visualization with reducing cerebral perfusion. In most settings, maintenance of normotension is recommended to prevent watershed injuries and may require blood transfusion and cardiovascular support. To aid in this setting of hemorrhage, neurophysiologic monitoring is critical as somatosensory evoked potentials (SSEPs) can provide insight to cerebral hypoperfusion. Direct carotid compression in the neck can be employed to help reduce the volume of flow and give the team more time to work. This can be augmented with a cervical incision and dissection to the carotid sheath. Anesthesia can provide temporary asystole (with adenosine) in order to help the surgical team visualize the injury and apply more direct control measures. Heparin infusion can also be considered to prevent embolic phenomena [5]. Constant communication with the anesthesiology team to replete blood products, administer drugs and avoid hypotension is paramount.

The size and type of the vascular injury is important in its management strategy. Once the bleeding has been temporized, the surgical team can work toward more definitive closure while simultaneously mobilizing the interventional neuroradiology team. Every attempt should be made to achieve a stable closure and avoid large volumes of subarachnoid blood and overall blood loss. Achieving proximal and distal vascular control may be challenging. Proximal control can also be achieved transcervically, by vascular clips if adequate exposure is achieved or direct compression within the field. Distal control can be similarly challenging. Direct control of the injury can be attempted with bipolar cautery or vascular clips in small injuries. Bipolar cautery can help control feeding vessels although one must be cognizant of the ramifications of sacrificing the superior hypophyseal artery and other branches off the basilar artery and Circle of Willis. Even smaller vessel injury can often be controlled with warm saline (40 °C) irrigation alone or by gentle application of thrombin-soaked absorbable gelatin, microfibrillar collagen, or oxidize cellulose. Neurophysiologic monitoring of cortical and brainstem function can be helpful in situations where branches off the Circle of Willis and basilar perforators are at risk. Venous injury (i.e., cavernous sinus and basilar plexus) can result in brisk bleeding as well, but this can usually be controlled by directly injecting a hemostatic matrix, applying gentle pressure and/or using bipolar cautery to seal the venous opening. Care should be taken to avoid inadvertent injection of flowable packing into the lumen of the carotid artery as this will result in microemboli with catastrophic neurologic consequences. Any use of vascular clips should be done with caution, especially with multiple cranial nerves adjacent in the cavernous sinus. Suturing in the endonasal corridor remains a significant shortcoming of this approach. Maneuvering in this situation requires an experienced team who can maintain a clear operative field. In large injuries, direct pressure and tamponade is often the preferred option. The materials vary from thrombin-soaked absorbable gelatin, oxidize cellulose, cotton, or preferably crushed muscle [6]. Additional pledgets may also be required to aid in applying adequate pressure.

Prior to leaving the operating room, the team must consider dural closure. Ideally, the injured vessel will be repaired with material that is either absorbable or does not require removal. The dura can then be reconstructed with grafting material or vascularized flaps. Once the sinonasal and intracranial compartments have been separated, additional absorbable and/or permanent packing (i.e., cottonoids or Merocels) can be placed. The decision to proceed immediately to the NeuroIR suite versus spending additional time achieving dural closure will depend on many factors including the patient's hemodynamics and any SSEP changes plus the readiness of the NeuroIR team. Additionally, the degree of vessel injury and types of materials used for initial reconstruction will play a role. Whether performed immediately or secondarily after NeuroIR, a sound dural closure will eventually be required.

Once hemostasis has been achieved, the patient is taken to the NeuroIR suite for an immediate angiogram and additional management as warranted. Once in the angiography suite, vessel patency can be assessed as can distal perfusion. The injured segment of the carotid artery can be reconstructed with a covered stent; however, vessel sacrifice with or without bypass may be required. Extrapolating from endarterectomy data, most patients will tolerate the sacrifice of one ICA [7]. A preoperative balloon test occlusion (BTO) can be valuable to help with decision making in this situation. Once stabilized, patients who suffer vascular injury should get a head CT to evaluate for intracranial hemorrhage. If the dura was not closed or pledgets were left in situ in order to facilitate expeditious transfer to angiography, the patient may require a return to OR. Postoperative epistaxis should be immediately investigated and may require imaging, repeat angiography, or a return to the OR. Lastly, all patients with an internal carotid artery injury should undergo an interval vascular evaluation to evaluate for possible formation of pseudoaneurysm.

References

1. Padhye V, Valentine R, Wormald PJ. Management of carotid artery injury in endonasal surgery. Int Arch Otorhinolaryngol. 2014;18(Suppl 2):S173–8.
2. Wang EW, et al. ICAR: endoscopic skull-base surgery. Int Forum Allergy Rhinol. 2019;9(S3):S145–365.
3. Gardner PA, et al. Carotid artery injury during endoscopic endonasal skull base surgery: incidence and outcomes. Neurosurgery. 2013;73(2 Suppl Operative):ons261–9; discussion ons269–70.
4. Wang WH, et al. The foramen lacerum: surgical anatomy and relevance for endoscopic endonasal approaches. J Neurosurg. 2018:1–12. https://doi.org/10.3171/2018.6.JNS181117.
5. Solares CA, et al. Prevention and management of vascular injuries in endoscopic surgery of the sinonasal tract and skull base. Otolaryngol Clin N Am. 2010;43(4):817–25.
6. Valentine R, Wormald PJ. Controlling the surgical field during a large endoscopic vascular injury. Laryngoscope. 2011;121(3):562–6.
7. Plestis KA, et al. Continuous electroencephalographic monitoring and selective shunting reduces neurologic morbidity rates in carotid endarterectomy. J Vasc Surg. 1997;25(4):620–8.

Part IV
Perioperative Management Related

Chapter 21
Complications Associated with Balloon Use

Mohamad R. Chaaban

Clinical Pearls

1. Balloon catheter dilation is a safe minimally invasive procedure with rare major complications. Otolaryngologists should carefully review the preoperative CT scan to examine the sinus/skull base anatomy and detect orbital or skull base dehiscence. All potential risks of BCD should be discussed with the patient along with the benefits of the procedure.
2. CSF leak following balloon catheter dilation is most commonly a result of frontal sinus dilation and should be surgically repaired intraoperatively at the time of the procedure. Delay in recognition or management may lead to severe neurological sequelae including meningitis, pneumocephalus, or brain abscess.
3. Orbital injuries with BCD may occur with maxillary sinus dilation leading to orbital wall fracture, pre/post septal orbital swelling or hematoma.

Case Presentation

A 65-year-old male with history of prior sinus surgery presented with persistent symptoms of sinus pressure and drainage. Following appropriate medical therapy, a preoperative CT scan showed an intact skull base. A planned left anterior ethmoidectomy, maxillary sinusotomy, and balloon frontal sinusotomy was performed. Confirmation of the wire entry into the frontal sinus was performed through forehead transillumination. The balloon was inflated to 12 cm H_2O and immediately following deflation, clear fluid was seen in the anterior ethmoid. The lateral lamellar

M. R. Chaaban (✉)
Head and Neck Institute, Cleveland Clinic, Cleveland, OH, USA
e-mail: chaabam@ccf.org

R. K. Chandra, K. C. Welch (eds.), *Lessons Learned from Rhinologic Procedure Complications*, https://doi.org/10.1007/978-3-030-75323-8_21

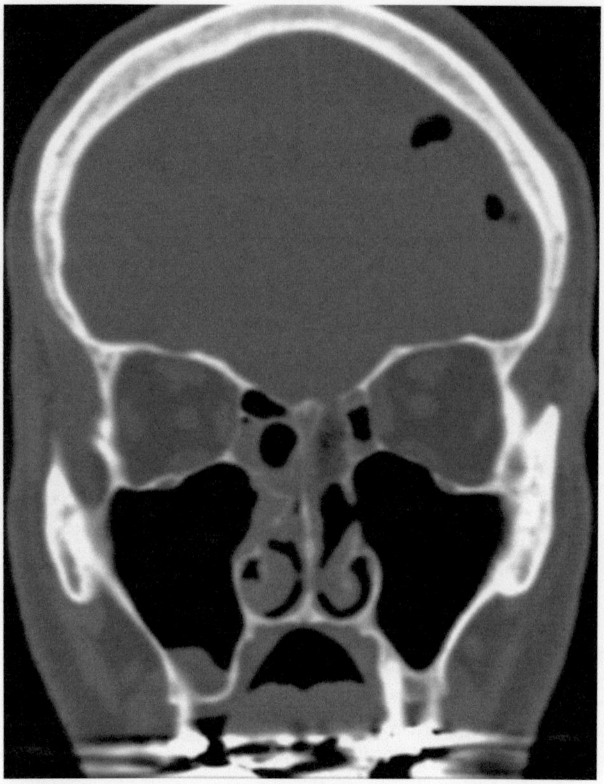

Fig. 21.1 Postoperative CT scan demonstrating a ~2 mm defect in the left lateral lamella of the cribriform. Pneumocephalus is also seen in the left cerebral hemisphere. (Reprinted with permission from reference [1])

defect was then repaired using an overlay graft and the patient was admitted for conservative management of CSF leak. Postoperative CT scan demonstrated the location of the defect in the left cribriform (Fig. 21.1) [1].

Root Cause Analysis

This case is an example of an intraoperative CSF leak in a patient that had no risk factors other than a prior sinus surgery, which may have led to scarring or loss of anatomical landmarks [2]. CSF leak following BCD can either be secondary to a perforation or a crack in the skull base. A perforation occurs when the catheter/balloon or an instrument is inadvertently inserted intracranially. The small size of the defect in this case (~2 mm) appears to most likely be a result of a crack either from direct pressure exerted directly or transmitted by the balloon during dilation. In the few other reported cases that included intraoperative findings, CSF leaks following BCD appear to occur at the lateral lamella of the cribriform [3, 4].

Lessons Learned

There are several risk factors that may lead to skull base injury during frontal sinus dilation (Table 21.1) [3, 5–8]. Prior to performing the procedure, the otolaryngologist should carefully review the CT scan to examine the depth of the skull base and frontal recess anatomy in relation to the frontal recess cells, and to look for a dehiscent skull base. Keros type 3 classification (olfactory fossa depth > 7 mm) was found to be higher in patients that developed iatrogenic CSF leaks (41%) compared to its incidence when it was initially described (18%) [5–7]. For physicians that rely on light confirmation instead of image guidance to confirm entry into the frontal sinus, it is prudent to look for the characteristic strong pinpoint light as opposed to dim light. A dim light may indicate that the wire is inserted in another cell such as a well-pneumatized supraorbital ethmoid. The otolaryngologist should also not force the balloon into the sinus if he/she is meeting resistance.

Complications in Balloon Catheter Dilation

Balloon catheter dilation (BCD) cleared the U.S. Food and Drug Administration (FDA) 510(k) pathway in 2005 as a minimally invasive sinus surgery. BCD has become an attractive option compared to conventional functional endoscopic sinus surgery (FESS) due to its less invasive nature. It can be used as a stand-alone procedure or combined with FESS as a hybrid procedure. Since its introduction, there has been an increase in the use of BCD as a stand-alone procedure from 5% in 2011 to 22.5% in 2014 [9].

Most of the prospective studies in the literature, including the clinical evaluation to confirm safety and efficacy of BCD in the paranasal sinuses (CLEAR study), reported little or zero adverse patient outcomes [10–17]. Despite the reported safety, complications from BCD can still occur and include minor and major complications. Major complications include severe bleeding, orbital hematoma, and skull base injury (CSF leak and pneumocephalus). The analysis of large administrative

Table 21.1 Risk factors associated with increased risk of CSF leak following balloon catheter dilation

Improper technique
Dehiscent skull base
Creation of a false passage (wire, catheter or balloon)
Revision surgery (scarring, loss of landmarks, and bony partitions)
Anatomical variants (Keros 3)
Bloody field
Hybrid procedure [3, 8]

health data from the Clinformatics Data Mart (CDM) database, one of the nation's largest commercial health insurance programs, the overall (minor and major) complication rate of BCD was 5.25% [18]. Orbital complications were most common at 2.95%, followed by bleeding at 2.03%, and skull base complication at 0.35% [18]. In this study, image guidance was not found to be protective against complications from sinus surgery.

An OpenFDA database, an online platform launched in 2014, contains information reported by physicians and manufacturers to the FDA [19]. Using this interface, Prince et al. reported an average of 12.6 annual adverse events (2006–2014) from BCD [20]. In the aforementioned study, the most common reported adverse events were patient injury ($n = 72$), followed by device failure (36), and death ($n = 4$). The most common reported patient injuries included orbital injuries ($n = 67$), skull base injuries ($n = 17$), and severe epistaxis ($n = 7$). A more recent study using the same OpenFDA database, by Wright et al. reported an average of 19.5 adverse events per year between 2015 and 2018 [2]. The increased reporting of adverse events may simply be due to the increase in use of BCD. In this recent study, the most common complications associated with BCD were device malfunction ($n = 44$), followed by patient injury ($n = 28$), and both ($n = 6$). Device malfunction was reported as balloon rupture (27%), which was associated with frontal sinus dilation, followed by device fracture (14%) and retention (14%).

Patient injuries from BCD can be broadly divided into local and systemic injuries. Systemic injuries include the very rare occurrence of arrhythmias or cardiac arrest [3, 21]. Local complications are usually dependent on the sinus dilated [2, 18, 20]. Skull base injuries and CSF leaks are reported with frontal sinus dilations, severe epistaxis with sphenoid-related dilations, and orbital wall fractures or pre/post septal orbital injuries with maxillary sinus dilations.

For CSF leaks, intraoperative detection and repair is the best approach to manage these complications. A delay in diagnosis of CSF leak may lead to untoward neurological sequelae such as pneumocephalus, intracranial hemorrhage, and ascending infection resulting in meningitis or brain abscess [3, 4, 22, 23]. The risk of death in patients that develop meningitis has been reported to occur as high as 37%, with permanent sequelae, in survivors, as high as 30% [24]. In a meta-analysis, early endoscopic repair of skull base defects resulted in a decrease in the risk of meningitis to 0.3% annually [25]. Unfortunately, in the OpenFDA reported complications, the timing of diagnosis of CSF leaks following BCD was not clear. However, the review of the individual reported cases of CSF leak secondary to BCD in the literature, most of them were diagnosed late [1–4].

Other major complications of BCD include severe epistaxis and orbital injury. Severe epistaxis may occur as a result of traumatizing the posterior septal branch of the sphenopalatine artery. Theoretical risks that are associated with sphenoid sinus dilations include injuries to dehiscent carotid artery or optic nerve, particularly if the balloon is inserted too deep into the sinus. It is crucial to review the CT scan preoperatively to look for carotid artery or optic nerve dehiscence. Orbital complications may occur with maxillary sinus dilations when either the balloon fractures the bony orbital wall or when the wire/catheter is inserted into a dehisced medial orbital wall. Fracture of the orbital wall may lead to periorbital swelling (Figs. 21.2 and 21.3) or hematoma [26].

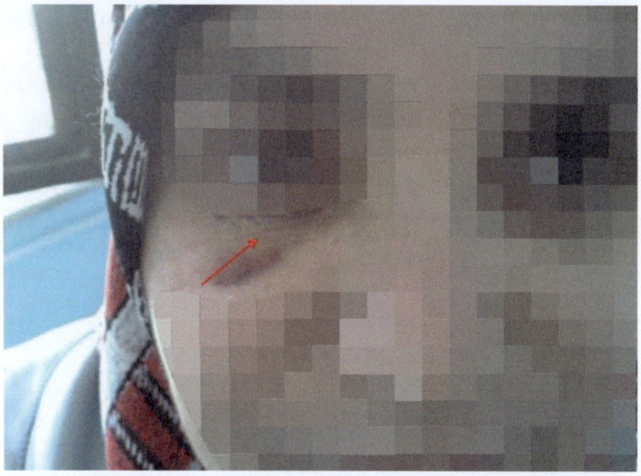

Fig. 21.2 Postoperative appearance of the patient 7 days following right maxillary BCD. Note that the patient had severe postoperative periorbital swelling that necessitated a subciliary incision for drainage. The patient recovered with no visual sequelae. (Reprinted with permission from reference [26])

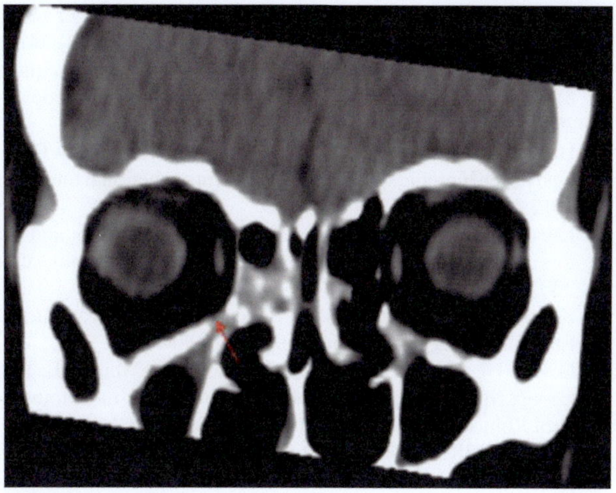

Fig. 21.3 Postoperative CT scan in the same patient demonstrating a fracture of inferomedial orbital wall. (Reprinted with permission from reference [26])

Sinus surgeries have consistently held one of the highest percentage of malpractice claims in the field of otolaryngology [10] with orbital and skull base injuries reported as the most common causes of malpractice litigation [27, 28]. Many of these stem from either negligent technique or lack of informed consent [28]. It is, therefore, imperative that otolaryngologists follow the guidelines on the appropriate use of this technology and discuss the risks candidly with the patients prior to the procedure. The worst outcome one would expect from BCD is a complication in a patient that should not have had the procedure in the first place. The published guidelines by American Academy of Otolaryngology – Head and Neck Surgery found no distinction between the indicated utilization of BCD and FES [29]. The clinical consensus statement on the use of BCD had several statements reaching consensus particularly in regards to the requirement of a CT scan prior to any BCD case [30]. In addition, BCD is not appropriate for patients with nasal polyps, headache, or sleep apnea, who do not meet the criteria for CRS or recurrent acute sinusitis [30].

Given the increasing popularity of BCD and the fact that this procedure is predominantly performed in the office [9], discussing the complications with the patients is of paramount importance. Otolaryngologists need to balance the risks associated with this minimally invasive procedure with the benefits of addressing symptoms of chronic rhinosinusitis, and meeting patients' expectations.

References

1. Sayal NR, Keider E, Korkigian S. Visualized ethmoid roof cerebrospinal fluid leak during frontal balloon sinuplasty. Ear Nose Throat J. 2018;97(8):E34–8.
2. Wright AE, Davis ED, Khan M, Chaaban MR. Exploring balloon sinuplasty adverse events with the innovative openFDA database. Am J Rhinol Allergy. 2020;34(5):626–31.
3. Tomazic PV, Stammberger H, Koele W, Gerstenberger C. Ethmoid roof CSF-leak following frontal sinus balloon sinuplasty. Rhinology. 2010;48(2):247–50.
4. Kubik M, Lee S, Snyderman C, Wang E. Neurologic sequelae associated with delayed identification of iatrogenic skull base injury during endoscopic sinus surgery (ESS). Rhinology. 2017;55(1):53–8. https://doi.org/10.4193/Rhin16.169.
5. Heaton CM, Goldberg AN, Pletcher SD, Glastonbury CM. Sinus anatomy associated with inadvertent cerebrospinal fluid leak during functional endoscopic sinus surgery. Laryngoscope. 2012;122:1446–9.
6. Lee JC, Song YJ, Chung YS, Lee BJ, Jang YJ. Height and shape of the skull base as risk factors for skull base penetration during endoscopic sinus surgery. Ann Otol Rhinol Laryngol. 2007;116:199–205.
7. Keros P. Uber die praktische Bedeutung der Niveauunterschiede der Lamina cribrosa des Ethmoid. Z Laryngol Rhinol. 1965;41:808–9.
8. Levine HL, Sertich AP 2nd, Hoisington DR, Weiss RL, Pritikin J, PatiENT Registry Study Group. Multicenter registry of balloon catheter sinusotomy outcomes for 1,036 patients. Ann Otol Rhinol Laryngol. 2008;117:263–70.
9. Chaaban MR, Baillargeon JG, Baillargeon G, Resto V, Kuo YF. Use of balloon sinuplasty in patients with chronic rhinosinusitis in the United States. Int Forum Allergy Rhinol. 2017;7(6):600–8.
10. Dawson DE, Kraus EM. Medical malpractice and rhinology. Am J Rhinol. 2007;21(5):584–90.
11. Kuhn FA, Church CA, Goldberg AN, Levine H, Sillers M, Vaughan W, Weiss R. Balloon catheter sinusotomy: one-year follow-up-outcomes and role in functional endoscopic sinus surgery. Otolaryngol Head Neck Surg. 2008;139(suppl):S27–37.
12. Weiss RL, Church CA, Kuhn FA, Levine HL, Sillers MJ, Vaughan WC. Long-term outcome analysis of balloon catheter sinusotomy: two-year follow-up. Otolaryngol Head Neck Surg. 2008;139(suppl):S38–46.
13. Ramadan HH. Safety and feasibility of balloon sinuplasty for treatment of chronic rhinosinusitis in children. Ann Otol Rhinol Laryngol. 2009;118(3):161–5.
14. Ramadan HH, Bueller H, Hester ST, Terrell AM. Sinus balloon catheter dilation after adenoidectomy failure for children with chronic rhinosinusitis. Arch Otolaryngol Head Neck Surg. 2012;138(7):635–7.
15. Ramadan HH, McLaughlin K, Josephson G, Rimell F, Bent J, Parikh SR. Balloon catheter sinuplasty in young children. Allergy Rhinol (Providence). 2010;1(2):11.
16. Ramadan HH, Terrell AM. Balloon catheter sinuplasty and adenoidectomy in children with chronic rhinosinusitis. Ann Otol Rhinol Laryngol. 2010;119(9):578–82.

17. Soler ZM, Rosenbloom JS, Skarada D, Gutman M, Hoy MJ, Nguyen SA. Prospective, multicenter evaluation of balloon sinus dilation for treatment of pediatric chronic rhinosinusitis. Int Forum Allergy Rhinol. 2017;7(3):221–9.
18. Chaaban MR, Rana N, Baillargeon J, Baillargeon G, Resto V, Kuo YF. Outcomes and complications of balloon and conventional functional endoscopic sinus surgery. Am J Rhinol Allergy. 2018;32(5):388–96.
19. Kass-Hout TA, Xu Z, Mohebbi M, Nelsen H, Baker A, Levine J, Johanson E, Bright R. OpenFDA: an innovative platform providing access to a wealth of FDA's publicly available data. J Am Med Inform Assoc. 2016;23(3):596–600.
20. Prince A, Bhattacharyya N. An analysis of adverse event reporting in balloon sinus procedures. Otolaryngol Head Neck Surg. 2016;154(4):748–53.
21. Hughes N, Bewick J, Van Der Most R, O'Connell M. A previously unreported serious adverse event during balloon sinuplasty. BMJ Case Rep. 2013;2013:bcr2012007879.
22. Krings JG, Kallogjeri D, Wineland NKG, Piccirillo JF, Getz AE. Complications of primary and revision functional endoscopic sinus surgery for chronic rhinosinusitis. Laryngoscope. 2013;124:838–45.
23. Stankiewicz JA, Lal D, Connor M. Complications in endoscopic sinus surgery for chronic rhinosinusitis: a 25 year experience. Laryngoscope. 2011;121:2684–90.
24. van de Beek D, Gans J, Tunkel A, et al. Community acquired bacterial meningitis in adults. N Engl J Med. 2006;354(1):44–53.
25. Hegazy HM, Carrau RL, Synderman CH, Kassam A, Zweig J. Transnasal endoscpic repair of cerebrospinal fluid rhinorrhea: a meta-analysis. Laryngoscope. 2000;110:1166–72.
26. Özkiriş M, Akin İ, Özkiriş A, Aydin R, Saydam L. Orbital complication of balloon sinuplasty. J Craniofac Surg. 2014;25(2):499–501.
27. Lynn-Macrae AG, Lynn Macrae RA, Emani J, Kern RC, Conley DB. Medicolegal analysis of injury during endoscopic sinus surgery. Laryngoscope. 2004;114:1492–5.
28. Shah SN, Ramirez AV, Haroun KB, Chaaban MR. Medical liability in sinus surgery: a Westlaw database analysis from 2000 to 2017. Am J Rhinol Allergy. 2020;34(5):642–9.
29. Rosenfeld RM, Piccirillo JF, Chandrasekhar SS, Brook I, Ashok Kumar K, Kramper M, Orlandi RR, Palmer JN, Patel ZM, Peters A, Walsh SA, Corrigan MD. Clinical practice guideline (update): adult sinusitis. Otolaryngol Head Neck Surg. 2015;152(4):598–609.
30. Piccirillo JF, Payne SC, Rosenfeld RM, Baroody FM, Batra PS, DelGaudio JM, Edelstein DR, Lane AP, Luong AU, Manes RP, McCoul ED, Platt MP, Reh DD, Corrigan MD. Clinical consensus statement: balloon dilation of the sinuses. Otolaryngol Head Neck Surg. 2018;158(2):203–14.

Chapter 22
Middle Turbinate Lateralization

Tran B. Locke and David W. Kennedy

Clinical Pearls

1. Middle turbinate lateralization occurs in a quarter of patients undergoing ESS. Avoiding intraoperative trauma to the middle turbinate minimizes the risk of lateralization and scarring.
2. Options to help prevent middle turbinate lateralization include absorbable or nonabsorbable packing used as a middle meatal spacer, middle turbinate–septal suture medialization, or creating a deliberate adhesion between the middle turbinate and nasal septum.
3. In the postoperative period, careful endoscopic examination and frequent debridement can help manage inflammatory foci and regions where synechiae formation could compromise results.

Case Presentation

A 72-year-old female presented with a history of multiple previous endoscopic sinus surgeries who was evaluated by an outside otolaryngologist for a soft tissue mass within the right frontal recess. Her primary complaints were excessive tearing, progressive blurry vision, occasional diplopia when looking down, and headache.

T. B. Locke
Department of Otolaryngology – Head and Neck Surgery, Baylor College of Medicine, Houston, TX, USA

D. W. Kennedy (✉)
Department of Otorhinolaryngology – Head and Neck Surgery, University of Pennsylvania, Philadelphia, PA, USA
e-mail: David.Kennedy@pennmedicine.upenn.edu

R. K. Chandra, K. C. Welch (eds.), *Lessons Learned from Rhinologic Procedure Complications*, https://doi.org/10.1007/978-3-030-75323-8_22

The otolaryngologist attempted to biopsy the mass intraoperatively but was unable to gain adequate exposure.

The patient was then referred to the University of Pennsylvania. Repeat CT scan demonstrated interval increase in size of the mass within the right frontal recess with erosion of the superior orbital roof, inferomedial lamina papyracea, and posterior table (Fig. 22.1). An MRI was performed that demonstrated a crescentic T2 hypointense lesion within the right ethmoid cavity, suggestive of a right frontal mucocele (Fig. 22.2).

During this time, her visual symptoms worsened, and decision was made to proceed with surgery. Intraoperatively, both middle turbinates were noted to be scarred to the lateral nasal wall along their longitudinal axes. The surrounding mucosa was inflamed, and the bone was osteitic, including the anterior portion of both middle turbinates. The overlying bone was meticulously taken down and the lining of the right frontal mucocele was incised and decompressed. The scar tissue within the left ethmoid cavity was similarly dissected out and the frontal recess widened (Fig. 22.3).

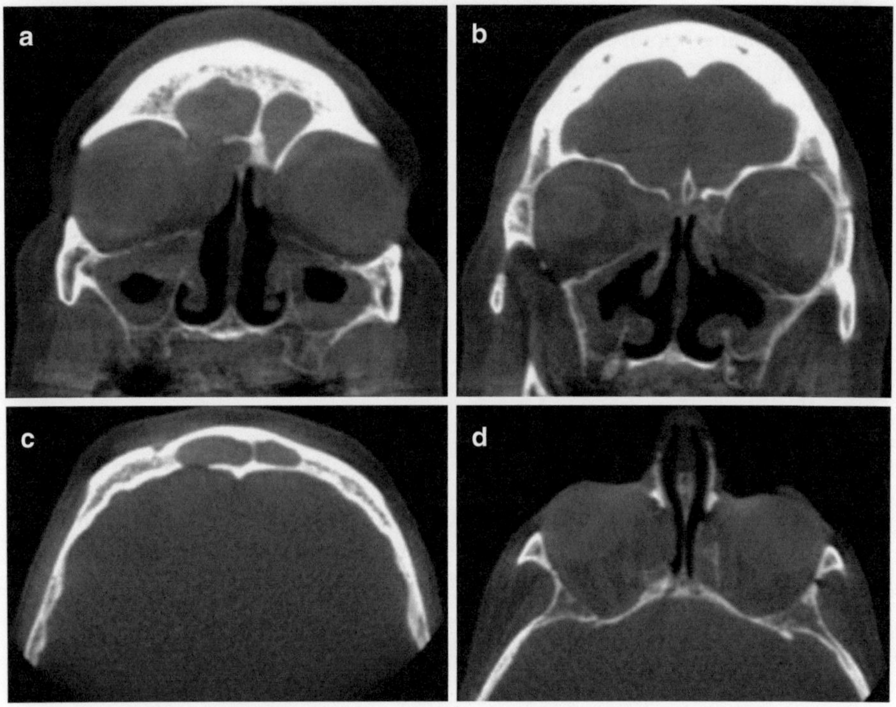

Fig. 22.1 Coronal (**a** and **b**) and axial (**c** and **d**) CT scan demonstrating bilateral opacification of the frontal sinuses with bony erosion of the right superior orbital roof, lamina papyracea, and posterior frontal table

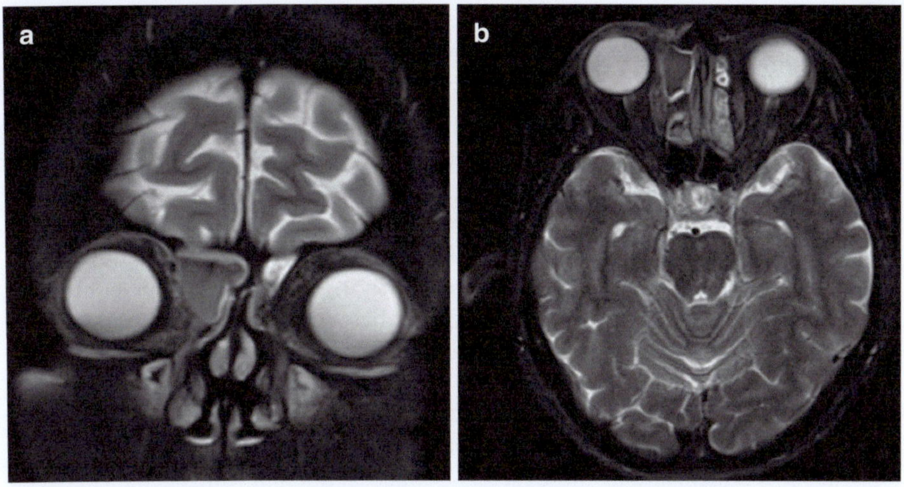

Fig. 22.2 T2-weighted coronal (**a**) and axial (**b**) MRI demonstrating bilateral opacification of the anterior ethmoid and frontal sinuses with a T2 hypointense lesion in the inferior right ethmoid bed, suggestive of adhesion or scar tissue

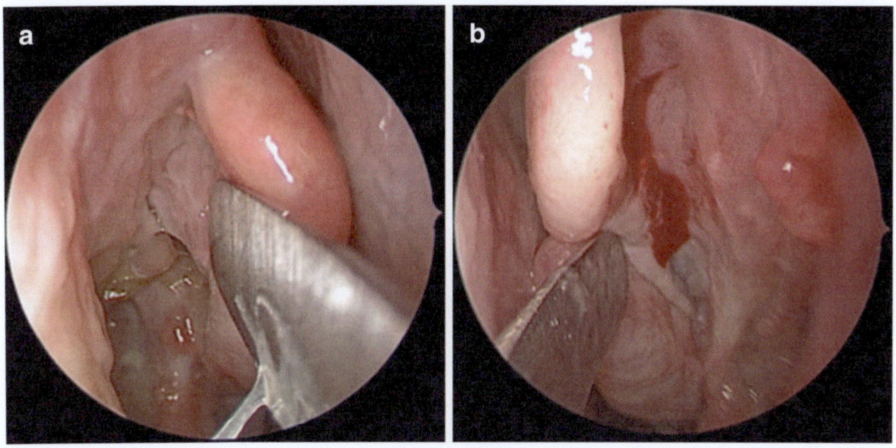

Fig. 22.3 (**a**) Lateralization of the right middle turbinate due to remnant superior uncinate; (**b**) lateralization of the left middle turbinate to the lateral nasal wall

To prevent recurrent lateralization of the middle turbinate, a small steroid-eluting stent was placed in the left ethmoid cavity.

Root Cause Analysis

The purpose of endoscopic sinus surgery (ESS) for medically recalcitrant chronic rhinosinusitis is to open the sinuses and allow for optimal aeration and delivery of topical medical therapies. However, postoperative complications such as adhesions, synechiae, and polyps can lead to unsatisfactory results. Of these complications, lateralization of the middle turbinate occurs in up to a quarter of patients who undergo ESS [1, 2]. Middle turbinate lateralization (MTL) with or without synechiae can form due to a number of factors such as destabilization of the middle turbinate from over-resection of the basal lamella or inadvertent mucosal trauma. The natural sequelae of trauma and inflammation are adhesions. However, the tendency to form adhesions and mucoceles varies widely from patient to patient. In addition to the underlying level of inflammation and the amount of surgical trauma, other contributing factors include allergy, as well as chemical exposures and smoking. The most critical among these factors is mucosal trauma, which occurs between two opposing edges, such as when a residual uncinate process creates a scar band between the turbinate and the lateral nasal wall. Since the uncinate process is typically involved in the inflammatory process, it is important at surgery to ensure that it is completely removed, thereby reducing the likelihood of an anterior middle turbinate adhesion. MTL results in poor mucociliary clearance and suboptimal delivery of topical mediations. Over time, the chronic inflammation leads to soft tissue and bony remodeling with subsequent scarring of the frontal and ethmoid outflow tracts, eventually requiring revision ESS [3] (Figs. 22.1 and 22.2). Complications can arise such as chronic sinusitis and mucocele formation, although the latter may not become clinically evident for many years.

Lessons Learned

Although some MTL can occur in the absence of opposing mucosal trauma, adhesions are extremely unlikely in the absence of middle turbinate trauma. Therefore, avoidance of trauma to the middle turbinate is extremely important in the prevention of such scarring. When MTL does occur, scarring can be avoided with meticulous postoperative management. Inflammation within the middle meatus and sinuses can be minimized by suctioning blood clot and fibrinous material and dividing any early adhesion formation. The administration of oral steroids and high-dose, high-volume topical nasal steroids is particularly important in patients with nasal allergy who are especially prone to posttraumatic edema and scar formation. Postoperative infection should be identified, cultured, and appropriately treated. There is evidence that some absorbable hemostatic agents may increase the risk of scarring and are therefore best avoided whenever possible at surgery [4].

Studies have evaluated the clinical impact of MTL after endoscopic sinus surgery and in extended endonasal approaches [3, 5]. MTL was not associated with higher LM scores [5] or patient-reported symptoms but may lead to earlier need for revision surgery [3]. However, it is very important to remember that mucoceles may not develop or become symptomatic for many years. Various intraoperative techniques have been used to medialize the middle turbinate postoperatively, including middle meatal nasal spacers, partial turbinate resection, controlled synechiae formation, and middle turbinate–septal suturing.

Controversy remains over which method best addresses MTL. Several studies have evaluated and compared the various medialization techniques. For instance, Soler et al. examined clinical outcomes after middle turbinate resection [6]. Their study found no difference in quality of life outcomes between preservation and resection of the middle turbinates. However, patients who had middle turbinate resection had more severe disease at baseline and greater improvement in endoscopy and smell identification test scores after ESS. Another area of debate involves the use of absorbable versus nonabsorbable nasal packing. A retrospective study by Xu et al. showed no significant difference in reduction of postoperative synechiae between steroid-impregnated absorbable spacers and nonabsorbable spacers [7]. A systematic review by Zhao et al. evaluated nonabsorbable, absorbable, and steroid-impregnated spacers and found no significant difference in synechiae formation if the nonabsorbable spacers were left in place for at least 48 h after surgery [2]. Another systematic review by Lee et al. showed that nonabsorbable spacers were more effective than absorbable spacers for reducing synechiae formation [4].

Other studies have demonstrated the effectiveness of middle turbinate–septal suture medialization as an alternative to nasal packing [8] or a combination of suture medialization and packing [1] to prevent MTL and improve postsurgical outcomes (Fig. 22.4).

When choosing a method, variables to consider include disease severity, available resources, patient disposition, and costs. Patients with severe recalcitrant disease, such as polypoid degeneration of the middle turbinate, may benefit from partial resection of the middle turbinate. The resources of the institution may dictate the type of spacers or packing used. Compared to standard absorbable or nonabsorbable packing, steroid-impregnated implants can be cost-prohibitive in some situations. Absorbable packing may be more desirable in certain patient circumstances, such as chronic anticoagulation or thrombocytopenia, low pain tolerance, or poor compliance. Packing markedly reduces the potential for suctioning inflamed mucus and pus in the early postoperative period, allowing for early resolution of inflammation. Accordingly, it is the senior author's practice to remove middle meatal sponges the day following surgery in most cases of inflammatory sinus disease.

Regardless of the intraoperative techniques used, efforts should be made to prevent MTL in the postoperative period.

In the postoperative period, adequate debridement and regular follow-up intervals with nasal endoscopy should be performed to ensure good healing and early recognition of scarring [9]. To help with postoperative edema and inflammation, all patients should be on a regimen consisting of nasal irrigations, typically with high-dose topical steroids added, routine sinus cavity debridement and careful

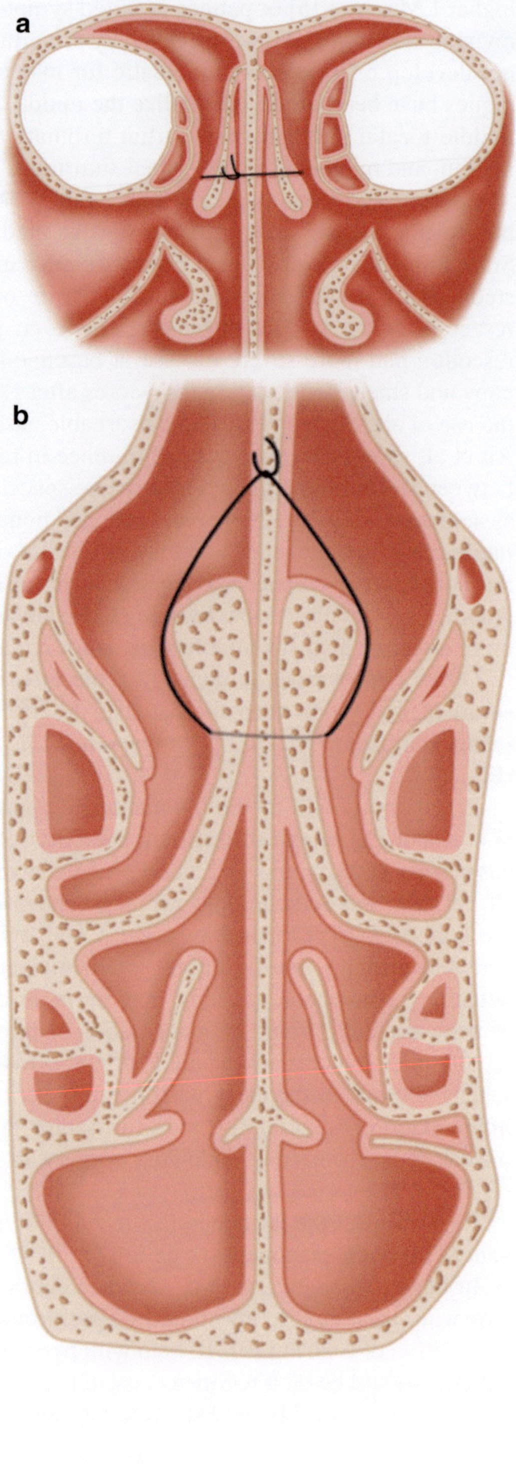

Fig. 22.4 Artist's depiction of suture medialization of bilateral middle turbinates. The technique can be combined with controlled mucosal abrasion of the medial aspect of the middle turbinates and the septum. (**a**) Coronal view. (**b**) Axial view

endoscopic follow-up for the potential for infection. Patients with marked inflammation, nasal polyposis, allergic diathesis, or allergic rhinitis should be placed on a steroid taper in the immediate postoperative period. Typically, 20–30 mg of prednisone (or equivalent) is sufficient to stabilize the nasal mucosa and may be tapered based upon the endoscopic findings. In-office lysis of synechiae or decompression of polypoid edema can reduce need for revision surgery. The debridement is aided by the use of targeted topical anesthesia (such as 4% cocaine or 4% pontocaine) on nasal applicators and, if necessary, localized injection of 1% Xylocaine with 1:100,000 epinephrine under endoscopic guidance. Other options following endoscopic sinus surgery include postoperative antibiotics, systemic steroids, and/or drug-eluting spacers/implants based on clinical judgment.

Advanced middle turbinate scarring may require more definitive surgical intervention as in the index case. In this situation, because the anterior portion of the middle turbinate was very osteitic, the turbinate was resected to the level of the frontal sinus. Although care was taken to minimize trauma and a steroid-eluting implant was used, there was still some tendency for the posterior portion of the middle turbinate to scar laterally. Given these factors, diligent postoperative management was performed. It is important to remember that patients who have previously formed a mucocele are at a significantly greater likelihood for reforming one. While the reasons for this are not totally clear, they may, at least in part, be related to allergy.

If there is persistent frontal sinus obstruction or mucocele formation, more extensive surgical management may be required in the form of a frontal sinus drill out (Draf 2B or Draf 3 procedure) or a frontal sinus rescue procedure. The frontal sinus rescue (FSR) procedure utilizes mucoperiosteal flap advancement in order to preserve the mucosa around the frontal ostium and frontal recess [10]. The FSR technique starts with a longitudinal incision along the middle turbinate remnant with subsequent elevation of the turbinate mucosa along its lateral and medial sides. The medial mucosa flap and bony turbinate remnant is removed up to the level of the skull base. The lateral mucoperiosteal flap is then draped medially, over the denuded area of the anterior nasal roof. This enlarges the frontal ostium and prevents scar contracture. A rolled Silastic stent is then used to hold the flap in position (Fig. 22.5).

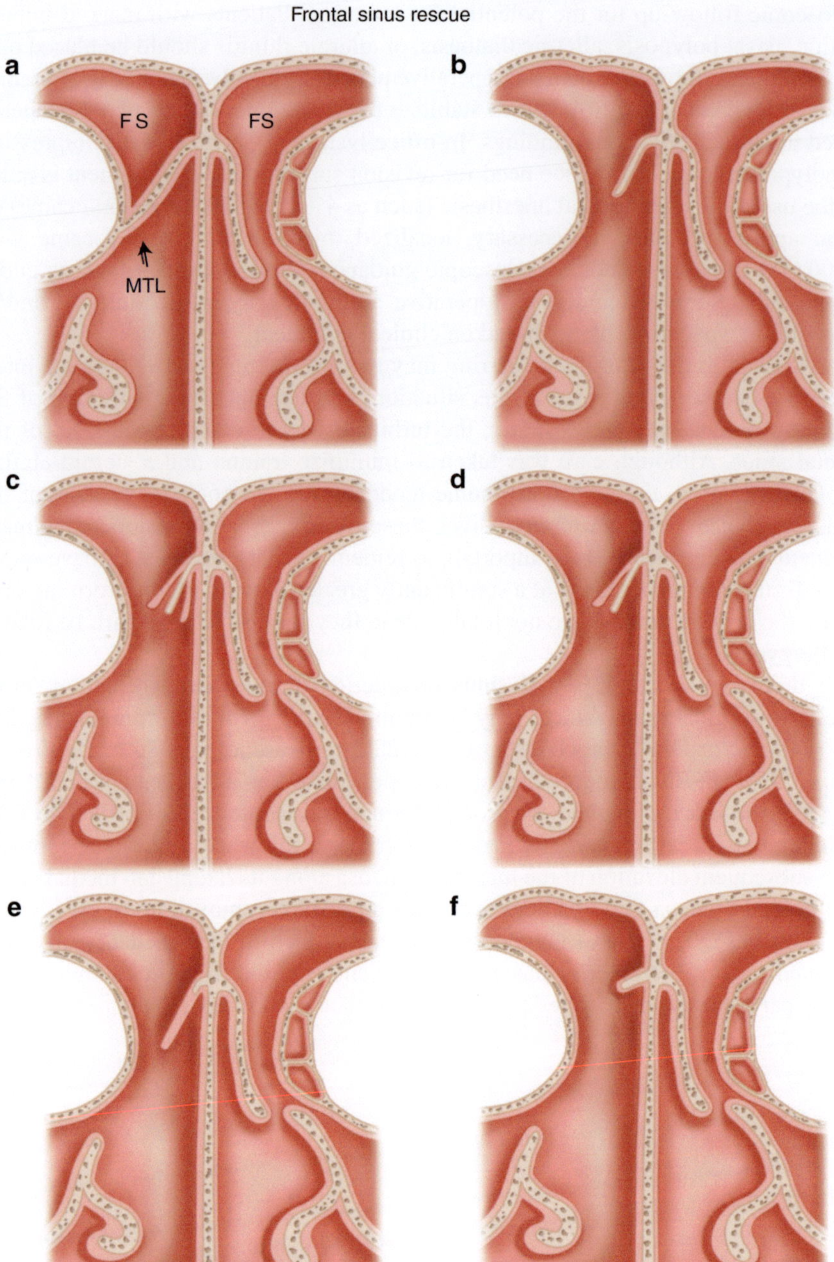

Fig. 22.5 Artist's depiction of frontal sinus rescue procedure. (**a**) The lateralized middle turbinate remnant (MTL) has blocked the frontal recess. (**b**) The lateral attachment of the middle turbinate is separated from the lamina. (**c**) The middle turbinate mucosa is elevated off the bone both laterally and medially. (**d**) The medial middle turbinate mucosal flap is removed as well as the adjacent septal mucosa. (**e**) The middle turbinate bony remnant is truncated, and the lateral middle turbinate mucosal flap is preserved. (**f**) The lateral middle turbinate mucosal flap is wrapped around the remaining bony middle turbinate attachment

Postoperative synechiae formation can lead to poorer outcomes after sinus surgery. Synechiae can occur anywhere in the sinuses, potentially leading to subsequent obstruction and a need for revision surgery. Middle turbinate lateralization and adhesions within the sinuses can be prevented through a number of intraoperative and postoperative strategies. The use of nonabsorbable middle meatal spacers, steroid-eluting implants, or suture medialization can help prevent MTL. Furthermore, careful endoscopic examinations and frequent debridement in the early postoperative period can ensure timely identification of problem areas and prevention of synechiae formation.

References

1. Chen W, Wang Y, Bi Y, Chen W. Turbinate-septal suture for middle turbinate medialization: a prospective randomized trial. Laryngoscope. 2015;125(1):33–5.
2. Zhao X, Grewal A, Briel M, Lee JM. A systematic review of nonabsorbable, absorbable, and steroid-impregnated spacers following endoscopic sinus surgery. Int Forum Allergy Rhinol. 2013;3(11):896–904.
3. Bassiouni A, Chen PG, Naidoo Y, Wormald PJ. Clinical significance of middle turbinate lateralization after endoscopic sinus surgery. Laryngoscope. 2015;125(1):36–41.
4. Lee JM, Grewal A. Middle meatal spacers for the prevention of synechiae following endoscopic sinus surgery: a systematic review and meta-analysis of randomized controlled trials. Int Forum Allergy Rhinol. 2012;2(6):477–86.
5. Willson TJ, Rowan NR, Wang EW. Middle turbinate manipulation and postoperative sinus obstruction after endoscopic endonasal skull-base surgery. Int Forum Allergy Rhinol. 2018;8(10):1132–5.
6. Soler ZM, Hwang PH, Mace J, Smith TL. Outcomes after middle turbinate resection: revisiting a controversial topic. Laryngoscope. 2010;120(4):832–7.
7. Xu JJ, Busato GM, McKnight C, Lee JM. Absorbable steroid-impregnated spacer after endoscopic sinus surgery to reduce synechiae formation. Ann Otol Rhinol Laryngol. 2016;125(3):195–8.
8. Hewitt KM, Orlandi RR. Suture medialization of the middle turbinates during endoscopic sinus surgery. Ear Nose Throat J. 2008;87(12):E11.
9. Rudmik L, Soler ZM, Orlandi RR, Stewart MG, Bhattacharyya N, Kennedy DW, et al. Early postoperative care following endoscopic sinus surgery: an evidence-based review with recommendations. Int Forum Allergy Rhinol. 2011;1(6):417–30.
10. Kuhn FA, Javer AR, Nagpal K, Citardi MJ. The frontal sinus rescue procedure: early experience and three-year follow-up. Am J Rhinol. 2000;14(4):211–6.

Chapter 23
Nasal Septum Perforation and Inferior Turbinate Avulsion/Unilateral Empty Nose Syndrome Resulting from Management of Recurrent Epistaxis

Angela Yang, Sachi Dholakia, Dayoung Kim, and Jayakar V. Nayak

Clinical Pearls

1. When treating septal causes of bleeding, judicious use of cautery on the nasal septum can help avoid creating septal perforations.
2. The ENS6Q, a validated and accepted questionnaire used to discriminate patients having empty nose syndrome (ENS) from other nasal conditions, can be used in the assessment of patients who are suspected to have ENS.
3. The Inferior Meatus Augmentation Procedure (IMAP) is a durable treatment option for augmentation of nasal tissues in patients with confirmed ENS.

Case Presentation

The patient is a 68-year-old male who reported a history of excellent health until 10 years ago, when he developed a cardiac/thromboembolic condition that required use of aspirin and clopidogrel for anticoagulation. In his first year of treatment, he unfortunately developed recurrent right-sided epistaxis. He recalled presenting to his local emergency department (ED) on multiple occasions to manage the nosebleeds, which led to multiple right-sided nasal cautery procedures. On his last ED visit, given profuse recurrent epistaxis, additional cautery of the nasal septum and right-sided nasal packing were pursued. Upon aggressive placement and advancement of the nasal packing into his right nasal cavity by the ED treatment team, the patient recalls experiencing an "unbearable, tearing sensation" and "excruciating, blistering pain" to his right face. Because of this traumatic experience, the patient

A. Yang · S. Dholakia · D. Kim · J. V. Nayak (✉)
Department of Otolaryngology – Head and Neck Surgery, Stanford University School of Medicine, Stanford, CA, USA
e-mail: jnayak@stanford.edu

R. K. Chandra, K. C. Welch (eds.), *Lessons Learned from Rhinologic Procedure Complications*, https://doi.org/10.1007/978-3-030-75323-8_23

was admitted and taken to the OR the following day by an otolaryngologist for additional surgical control of epistaxis. After this procedure, he learned that a large nasal septum perforation was found, and that "there was damage to his nasal turbinate" but that nothing further could be offered.

Since that event, the patient's nosebleeds never returned, and eventually his anticoagulant medications were discontinued. However, for the past 10 years, he acquired numerous new, bothersome issues regarding his nasal breathing, including whistling with inhalation, severe, continuous right nasal obstruction, right nasal burning, sensation of nasal pain with breathing, dry mouth, and formation of large crusts released weekly from the nose. He never experienced any left-sided nasal complaints. The patient sought help from multiple otolaryngologists, who offered limited treatment options, until he was referred to the Stanford Sinus Center for further management.

On nasal endoscopy, a 2.5 cm anterior septal perforation was noted. Moreover, complete loss of the right inferior turbinate, including the turbinate attachment to lateral wall, was noted (Fig. 23.1). Computed tomography (CT) imaging confirmed these striking findings (Fig. 23.2). Given the detailed and unusual history of severe, traumatic unilateral discomfort with packing placement, combined with these findings, the most likely explanation for these nasal findings was (1) tissue loss to the anterior septum due to repeated cauterizations and ischemia to the septum mucosa and cartilage; (2) complete avulsion of the right inferior turbinate upon aggressive placement of nasal packing, leading to right-sided empty nose syndrome (ENS) symptoms.

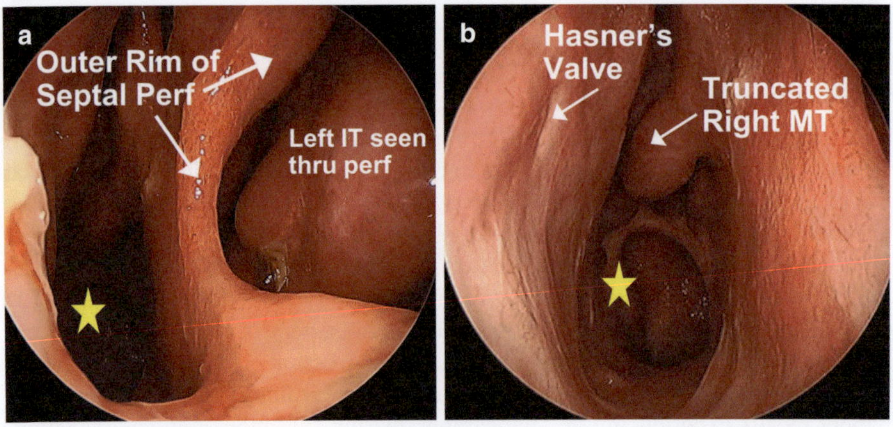

Fig. 23.1 Nasal endoscopy from right side of nose. (**a**) Widely patent right nasal cavity due to complete loss of the right inferior turbinate (yellow star), and perforation through the central nasal septum (rim of perforation is noted). The intact left inferior turbinate (IT) can be seen from the right nostril through the septal perforation. (**b**) Complete loss of the right IT after avulsion, with direct view of Hasner's valve, the middle turbinate (MT) remnant, and the choana of the nasopharynx

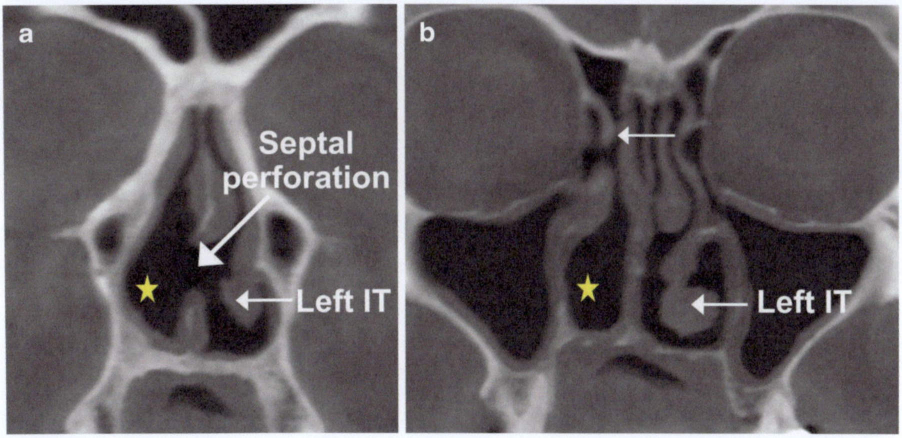

Fig. 23.2 Sinus CT, coronal views from the anterior (**a**), and central (**b**) nasal cavity. (**a**) Central septal perforation is labeled, and wide patency of the right nasal airway (yellow star). (**b**) Stark difference between the asymptomatic left nasal airway with normal inferior turbinate, and open right nasal airway, devoid of any features of the right inferior turbinate (star)

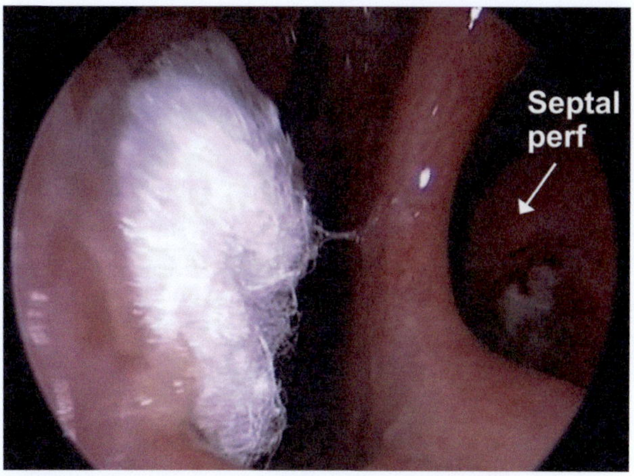

Fig. 23.3 Cotton test of right nasal airway. Dry, fashioned cotton plug placed in right inferior meatus to simulate right IT bulk and contour. This simple maneuver markedly improved the uncomfortable sensation associated with right-sided nasal airflow in this patient with complete IT soft tissue loss

On presentation, the patient completed the empty nose syndrome (ENS) 6-Item Questionnaire (ENS6Q), and scored 15 out of maximum 30 based solely on his right-sided symptoms. Given that a score of 0–5 is normal nasal breathing for the ENS6Q, and a score between 11 and 30 is considered positive, his score of 11 was strongly suggestive of ENS. In-office cotton test was performed, with dry cotton plug placement into the right inferior meatus (Fig. 23.3). Within 1 min following cotton placement, the patient reported significant improvement in his right nasal breathing, with reduced nasal burning and dry throat sensation. Repeat ENS6Q testing with cotton in situ demonstrated a drop in his subjective score to 3 out of 30, a reduction of 12 points in the cardinal symptoms of ENS. Given his

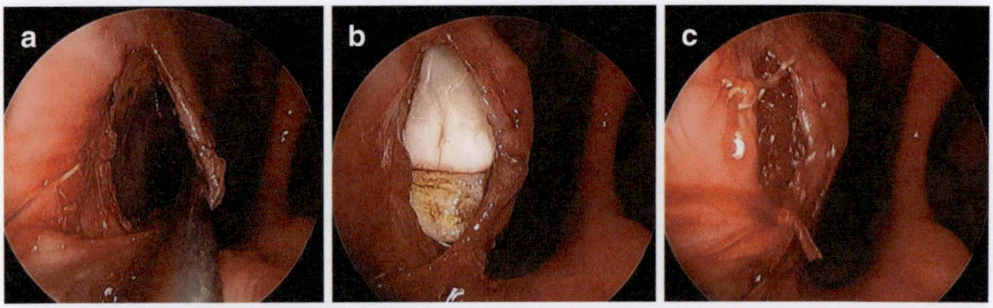

Fig. 23.4 Inferior meatus augmentation procedure (IMAP). (**a**) In the OR, a submucosal pocket is created at the right inferior meatus cavity. (**b**) Two pieces of cadaveric rib were placed in antiseptic, then whittled down, fashioned, and placed into the submucosal tunnel to create a neo-turbinate. This "speed bump" has excellent projection from the sidewall into the airway, and a tubular shape akin to the natural contour of the turbinate. (**c**) Gelfoam placed for hemostasis, with closure of submucosal access using resorbable suture

baseline ENS6Q score greater than 11 [1], and positive office cotton test with a drop of at least 7 points [2], the patient was formally diagnosed with right-sided ENS. He was recommended to undergo a unilateral, right-sided inferior meatus augmentation procedure (IMAP) using a fashioned cadaveric rib graft, which proceeded successfully (Fig. 23.4). Postoperatively, the patient reported complete resolution of all of his long-standing preoperative nasal symptoms, including improved nasal breathing and reduced nasal and throat discomfort. The postoperative ENS6Q scores at 1 month and 2 months were 0/30 and 1/30, respectively, and the patient was extremely pleased with his improved quality of life (QoL). The anterior nasal septum perforation was left intact given its large diameter, well-mucosalized borders, and lack of direct influence on this patient's nasal breathing.

Root Cause Analysis

Nasal septal perforations are commonly associated with trauma [3], intranasal drug use [4], or autoimmune diseases such as granulomatosis with polyangiitis (GPA) [5]. In this case, the etiology of the septal perforation was repeated use of chemical or electrocautery to control epistaxis, leading to tissue ischemia. From our review of the literature, no cases of septal perforation occurring through this mechanism could be identified. In this patient's rare case, the mechanism of turbinate loss is avulsion of the entire right turbinate during nasal packing placement for the management of his epistaxis. As nasal packing is known to cause pain and infectious complications, precise and careful placement of nasal packing is essential.

Lessons Learned

ENS is a complex syndrome first formally described in 1994 by Kern and Stenkvist when they recognized that some patients who underwent inferior or middle turbinate (IT or MT) surgery complained of nasal obstruction, dryness, and crusting [6]. Identification of ENS can be challenging as patients' nasal anatomy is objectively patent despite their complaints of obstruction, often termed paradoxical nasal obstruction. Typically, turbinate tissue loss occurs during turbinoplasty surgery, turbinate tissue loss, or turbinoplasty [6]. In this patient's rare case, the mechanism of turbinate loss is avulsion of the entire right turbinate during nasal packing placement. Nasal packing remains the most common management for epistaxis [7] due to the providing of pressure and tamponing to stop the bleed. Depending on location of packing placement, nasal packing is associated with both pain [8] and toxic shock syndrome [9].

The ENS6Q is a validated and widely accepted questionnaire used to discriminate patients having ENS from other nasal conditions. The questionnaire asks patients to subjectively rate the six major symptoms associated with ENS: "nasal dryness," "nose feels too open," "nasal suffocation," "sense of diminished airflow," "nasal crusting," and "nasal burning." A score of 11 out of 30 is considered clinically significant [1]. When a patient complains of a combination of the nasal symptoms above, physicians should consider ENS in the differential diagnosis. The patient's nasal surgical history and imaging should be reviewed, and the ENS6Q questionnaire can readily be administered Nasal endoscopy and/or cotton test should be performed prior to topical application of decongestants or anesthetics. If turbinate tissue loss is confirmed in a patient whose ENS6Q score is greater than, or equal to, 11, a cotton test should be performed. This provocation test is completed through unilateral or bilateral placement of dry cotton in plugs into the inferior meatal space (IM) to simulate the contour of the missing native turbinate tissue using cotton [10]. Patients with a decline of at least 7 points in their ENS6Q scoring, the minimal clinically important difference (MCID), is considered positive for ENS, and candidates for nonsurgical or surgical treatment [2].

Traditional nonsurgical treatment options include the use of nasal irrigations, emollients, topical antibiotics, nasal humidification, or topical steroids [10]. More recent studies have examined the influence of trigeminal retraining therapy on alleviating nasal obstruction and improving QoL [11].

Prior to offering surgical intervention, the use of intranasal submucosal fillers to augment the nasal tissues may be performed in the office setting. There are two main types of filler material in the literature – autologous stromal vascular fraction (SVF)/adipose-derived stem cells (ADSC), or use of inert, colloidal gel materials such as carboxymethylcellulose (CMC) or hyaluronic acid (HA) gel. While there is conflicting evidence on the benefit of SVF for ENS [12, 13], injection of gel fillers has been shown to transiently, but effectively, improve patients' symptoms and psychological parameters [14, 15]. These filler materials are slowly resorbed over several weeks/months, but if sustained beneficial effects are noted, these agents provide further credence of the diagnosis of ENS to both the patient and treating physician. Injection procedure protocols may vary depending on physicians, and the average time for the gel to resorb depends on the precise material and brand used. Often this resorbable gel filler injection is performed on patients with a borderline clinically significant ENS6Q score, or patients who have an equivocal response to the cotton test. Patients who benefit from filler injection into the IM may choose to proceed with additional rounds of injections (every 3–4 months), or consider surgical treatment for ENS.

The inferior meatus augmentation procedure (IMAP) [16] is a durable treatment option for augmentation of nasal tissues that requires general anesthesia. Common graft materials include small intestinal submucosa (SIS) graft, acellular dermal matrix [16, 17], or autologous versus cadaveric rib grafts. In a recent meta-analysis of six studies with a total of 122 ENS patients who underwent implant surgery, allograft was found to be more effective than foreign material grafts [18], and our own findings show an aggregate improvement/normalization in the pattern of nasal airflow in pre- versus post-IMAP CT imaging of ENS patients using computational fluid dynamics (CFD) modeling (J. V. Nayak, manuscript submitted).

If a patient presents with ENS-associated breathing complaints, but also has evidence of concurrent sinonasal disease such as chronic rhinosinusitis or fungal sinusitis, we recommend proceeding in a stepwise manner to first address the non-ENS, inflammatory, and/or infectious diseases burden. At a later date, once the major sinonasal disease is managed, the patient may be reassessed and retested for ENS. The latter plan of care eliminates all confounding sinonasal elements that may impact proper evaluation of ENS.

It should also be noted that many ENS patients have severely decreased QoL, are often handicapped from performing activities of daily living, and suffer from psychological burdens such as anxiety or depression [19, 20]. If the patient expresses suicidal ideation, however, the physician should always recommend an immediate referral to a mental health professional.

ENS remains a rare complication of nasal surgery and, currently, there is no consensus on the complication rate. As practitioners who see a high volume of patients with ENS, we estimate the rate of ENS to be between 1:750 and 1:1000 turbinoplasties performed. While the etiology of ENS is still unclear, the majority of cases are strongly linked to aggressive inferior turbinoplasty surgery and inferior turbinate resection, or suboptimal tissue healing after well-executed inferior turbinoplasty [21]. Additionally, it should be noted that sporadic cases of "middle turbinate ENS" have also been reported after middle turbinate resection [22]. In the case of this 68-year-old male, the patient sustained iatrogenic ENS caused by complete avulsion of his right inferior turbinate during nasal packing placement for epistaxis control. In addition, repeated cautery to the nasal septum also for control of epistaxis, likely led to iatrogenic ischemia/necrosis of the septal tissue, and a large anterior nasal septal perforation.

One increasingly substantiated hypothesis for the physiopathology of ENS is that altered turbinate tissue volume and contour results in aberrant airflow patterns.

In a study of six patients with confirmed ENS performed at Ohio State, post-IT reduction CT scans were analyzed using computational fluid dynamic (CFD) simulation and showed distorted nasal airflow that was concentrated as a jet stream toward the middle meatus region, compared to normal, healthy controls that show broadly distributed airflow between the inferior and middle meatuses [23]. Another theory is that because the trigeminal nerve is involved in the perception of nasal airflow, turbinate surgery may cause sensory damage, thereby diminishing the sense of airflow [24]. In a study comparing nasal trigeminal sensitivity, on average, the 27 ENS patients had impaired nasal trigeminal function as compared to 42 healthy controls [21].

In our opinion, to prevent a major segment of iatrogenic ENS, practitioners should aim to preserve the position and shape of the turbinate tissue, unless removal of the turbinate tissue is essential such as in the setting of malignancy. When reduction of the turbinate may be needed, such as recalcitrant soft tissue hypertrophy, it is advised to conservatively reduce the turbinate tissue caliber and volume while retaining the overall tubular shape of the turbinate. The risks of turbinate surgery should also be explained to the patient preoperatively.

References

1. Velasquez N, Thamboo A, Habib A-RR, Huang Z, Nayak JV. The Empty Nose Syndrome 6-Item Questionnaire (ENS6Q): a validated 6-item questionnaire as a diagnostic aid for empty nose syndrome patients. Int Forum Allergy Rhinol. 2017;7:64–71.
2. Thamboo A, et al. Defining surgical criteria for empty nose syndrome: validation of the office-based cotton test and clinical interpretability of the validated Empty Nose Syndrome 6-Item Questionnaire. Laryngoscope. 2017;127:1746–52.
3. Pereira C, et al. Nasoseptal perforation: from etiology to treatment. Curr Allergy Asthma Rep. 2018;18:5.
4. Lanier B, Kai G, Marple B, Wall GM. Pathophysiology and progression of nasal septal perforation. Ann Allergy Asthma Immunol. 2007;99:473–80.
5. Trimarchi M, et al. Otorhinolaryngological manifestations in granulomatosis with polyangiitis (Wegener's). Autoimmun Rev. 2013;12:501–5.
6. Sozansky J, Houser SM. Pathophysiology of empty nose syndrome. Laryngoscope. 2015;125:70–4.
7. Meccariello G, et al. Management of idiopathic epistaxis in adults: what's new? Acta Otorhinolaryngol Ital. 2019;39:211–9.
8. Womack JP, Kropa J, Stabile MJ. Epistaxis: outpatient management. Am Fam Physician. 2018;98:240–5.
9. Lange JL, Peeden EH, Stringer SP. Are prophylactic systemic antibiotics necessary with nasal packing? A systematic review. Am J Rhinol Allergy. 2017;31:240–7.
10. Chhabra N, Houser SM. The diagnosis and management of empty nose syndrome. Otolaryngol Clin N Am. 2009;42:311–30.
11. Bon S-DL, Horoi M, Bon OL, Hassid S. Intranasal trigeminal training in empty nose syndrome: a pilot study on 14 patients. Clin Otolaryngol. 2020;45:259–63.
12. Kim D-Y, Hong HR, Choi EW, Yoon SW, Jang YJ. Efficacy and safety of autologous stromal vascular fraction in the treatment of empty nose syndrome. Clin Exp Otorhinolaryngol. 2018;11:281–7.

13. Xu X, et al. The expansion of autologous adipose-derived stem cells in vitro for the functional reconstruction of nasal mucosal tissue. Cell Biosci. 2015;5:54.
14. Modrzyński M. Hyaluronic acid gel in the treatment of empty nose syndrome. Am J Rhinol Allergy. 2011;25:103–6.
15. Borchard NA, et al. Use of intranasal submucosal fillers as a transient implant to alter upper airway aerodynamics: implications for the assessment of empty nose syndrome. Int Forum Allergy Rhinol. 2019;9:681–7.
16. Thamboo A, et al. Inferior meatus augmentation procedure (IMAP) to treat empty nose syndrome: a pilot study. Otolaryngol Head Neck Surg. 2020;162:382–5.
17. Velasquez N, Huang Z, Humphreys IM, Nayak JV. Inferior turbinate reconstruction using porcine small intestine submucosal xenograft demonstrates improved quality of life outcomes in patients with empty nose syndrome. Int Forum Allergy Rhinol. 2015;5:1077–81.
18. Ma Z, Quan-Zeng, Jie-Liu, Hu G. Assessment of postsurgical outcomes between different implants in patients with empty nose syndrome: a meta-analysis. J Int Med Res. 2017;45:1939–48.
19. Manji J, Nayak JV, Thamboo A. The functional and psychological burden of empty nose syndrome. Int Forum Allergy Rhinol. 2018;8:707–12.
20. Lee T-J, et al. Evaluation of depression and anxiety in empty nose syndrome after surgical treatment. Laryngoscope. 2016;126:1284–9.
21. Malik J, et al. Computational fluid dynamic analysis of aggressive turbinate reductions: is it a culprit of empty nose syndrome? Int Forum Allergy Rhinol. 2019;9:891–9.
22. Houser SM. Empty nose syndrome associated with middle turbinate resection. Otolaryngol Head Neck Surg. 2006;135:972–3.
23. Li C, et al. Computational fluid dynamics and trigeminal sensory examinations of empty nose syndrome patients. Laryngoscope. 2017;127:E176–84.
24. Li C, et al. Investigation of the abnormal nasal aerodynamics and trigeminal functions among empty nose syndrome patients. Int Forum Allergy Rhinol. 2018;8:444–52.

Chapter 24
Stent Complications

Taylor R. Carle and Jeffrey D. Suh

Clinical Pearls

1. Ensure documentation of stent placement in the operative report, disclose stent use to the patient, and consider stent removal to reduce the risk of delayed stent complications. Periodic imaging should be considered for long-term stenting to assess for migration or malpositioning.
2. Postoperative ocular complaints should trigger concern for complication necessitating a comprehensive ocular evaluation, endoscopy, or imaging.
3. All sinus stents are comprised of foreign body material and thus run the risk of developing biofilms, infections, or hypersensitivity reactions. These adverse events can lead to recalcitrant sinusitis necessitating stent removal.

Case Presentation

A 43-year-old male with a history of chronic rhinosinusitis (CRS) had bilateral functional endoscopic sinus surgery (FESS) with placement of a Rains frontal sinus stent. Postoperatively he recovered well per the otolaryngologist's notes, with no unusual symptoms. Three months after the surgery he had a seizure while driving, lost consciousness, and had a motor vehicle accident. He was brought to the local Emergency Room for evaluation. In addition to multiple lacerations, he was found to have fractures of C2 and T12 vertebral bodies on imaging.

A CT and MRI of the brain and sinuses were also obtained, which revealed a frontal sinus stent traversing through the left ethmoid skull base into the anterior cranial fossa with a surrounding 2 cm frontal lobe abscess (Figs. 24.1 and 24.2). At

T. R. Carle · J. D. Suh (✉)
UCLA Department of Head and Neck Surgery, Los Angeles, CA, USA
e-mail: jeffsuh@mednet.ucla.edu

R. K. Chandra, K. C. Welch (eds.), *Lessons Learned from Rhinologic Procedure Complications*, https://doi.org/10.1007/978-3-030-75323-8_24

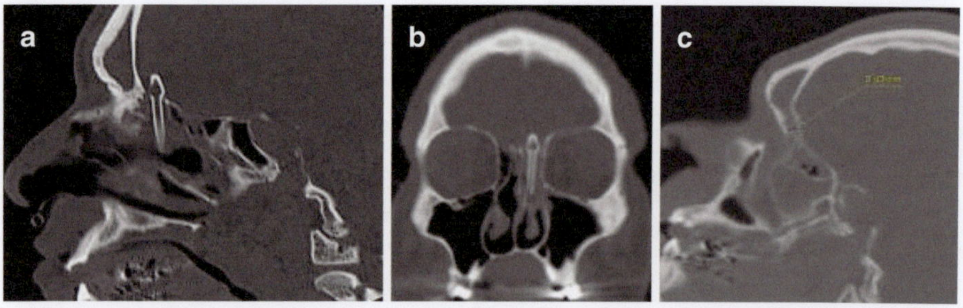

Fig. 24.1 CT sinus noncontrast scans showing (**a**) sagittal, (**b**) coronal views demonstrating the intracranial placement of the Rains frontal sinus stent into the anterior cranial fossa. The narrow anterior–posterior diameter of the frontal sinus outflow tract is demonstrated in a sagittal view in (**c**)

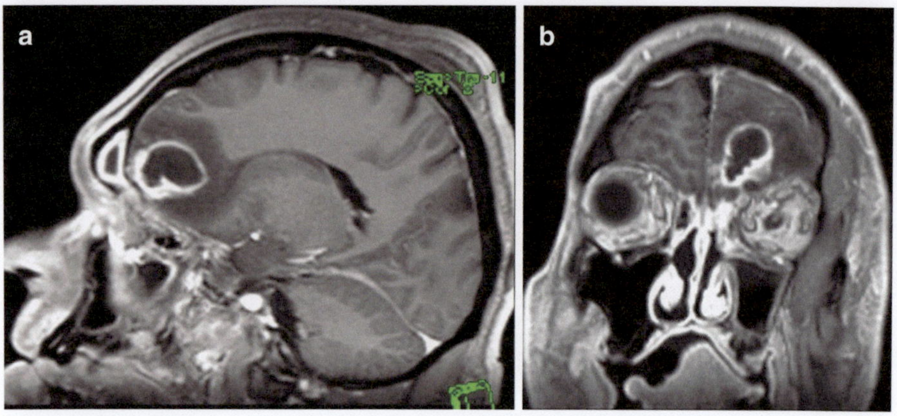

Fig. 24.2 T1-weighted MRI brain with contrast showing a left frontal lobe abscess in the (**a**) sagittal and (**b**) coronal views

that time, the patient was hemodynamically stable. He was placed in spinal precautions, started on IV antibiotics and transferred to our tertiary care hospital for surgical management.

The patient was taken to the operating room for stent removal, abscess drainage, and skull base reconstruction. The surgery was done endoscopically, with neurosurgery assistance for the abscess drainage. Of note, the patient had extremely complex frontal sinus anatomy with a small anterior–posterior distance in the frontal recess. A unilateral modification of the outside-in Draf 3 technique [1] was utilized to safely enter the frontal sinus first, then to identify the skull base. The frontal sinus was full of mucopurulence, which was sampled for culture analysis, then irrigated using antibiotic solution.

A Rains frontal sinus stent (Gyrus ACMI, Southborough, MA) was found penetrating through the fovea ethmoidalis just posterior to the left frontal sinus (Fig. 24.3). The stent was then carefully removed, and the abscess was drained through the defect. The skull base defect was approximately 2.5 cm in length × 1 cm

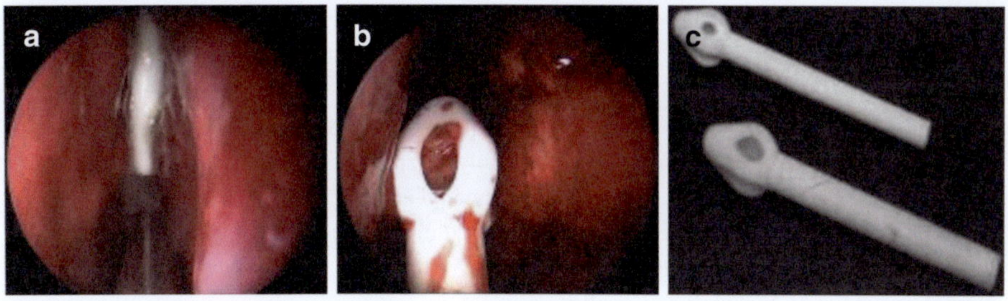

Fig. 24.3 Intraoperative demonstration of the Rains stent within the left nasal cavity (**a**) and following removal from the skull base defect (**b**). (**c**) Two sizes of Rains Frontal Sinus stents, 4 mm OD regular size (top) and 6 mm OD larger size (bottom)

Fig. 24.4 Postoperative imaging 6 months following surgery, demonstrating interval resolution of left frontal abscess on T2-weighted MRI brain with contrast

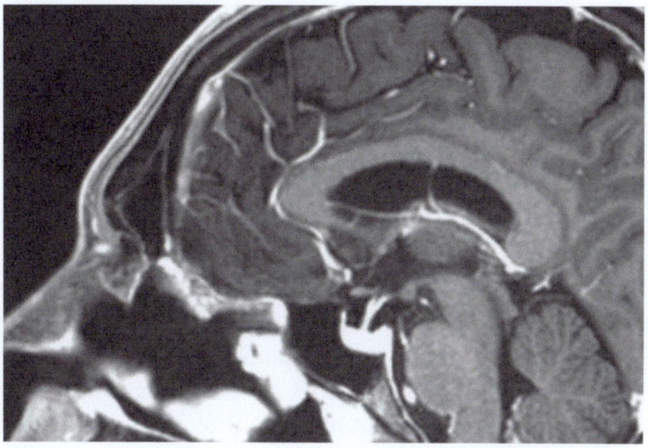

in width, and was reconstructed with a pedicled nasoseptal flap. Intraoperative cultures grew *Stenotrophomonas maltophilia*, *Staphylococcus epidermidis*, and *Streptococcus anginosis*.

The Infectious Disease service recommended a 6-week course of intravenous ceftazidime, metronidazole, and vancomycin. At the 3-week postoperative evaluation, the nasal packing and frontal sinus spacer were removed. Postoperative imaging obtained at 6 months revealed a well-healed skull base reconstruction and resolution of the intracranial infection (Fig. 24.4). Five years after the accident, the patient can ambulate without assistance, but still has some cognitive impairment.

Root Cause Analysis

Stents have been utilized in FESS to reduce the rate of surgical failure for decades. Many types of stents are commonly used in sinus surgery, made up of a wide variety of materials (Tables 24.1 and 24.2). More recently, drug-eluting stents have been introduced with excellent clinical results. The common goal of stent utilization is to

Table 24.1 Stent types and material

Stent name/ material	Material
Silastic	Synthetic polymer made up of silicon, oxygen, and other elements.
Propel	Synthetic bioabsorbable copolymer, poly (L-lactide-co-glycolide) (PLG)
Merocel	Polymer of hydroxylated polyvinyl acetate
Telfa	Absorbent cotton fibers enclosed in a sleeve of polyethylene terephthalate
Latex (natural)	Sap harvested from rubber trees
Nitinol	Nickel–titanium alloy
Teflon	Polytetrafluroethylene
Chitosan	Polysaccharide of β-(1→4)-linked D-glucosamine and N-acetyl-D-glucosamine.

Table 24.2 Stent types and names

Material	Examples
Silastic/silicone	Rains, Doyle splint, liberty bell
Poly (L-lactide-co-glycolide) (PLG)	Propel, mini, contour, Sinuva
Nitinol	ArchSinus
Chitosan	Hemopore, Chitogel, PosiSep

reduce the development of adhesions, ostial stenosis, mucosal inflammation, and middle turbinate lateralization [2–3]. These adverse events are the most common inciting factors for symptom recurrence and revision surgery [4]. Although rare, stents can also be associated with complications. These complications range from local reactions (granulation tissue, infection, dislocation, epistaxis, hypersensitivity reactions), to violation of nearby anatomic structures such as the skull base and orbit, to systemic reactions including toxic shock syndrome (TSS) [5–11].

Local Reaction and Hypersensitivity

Stents used in FESS are composed of a wide variety of materials. These stents, while generally inert, can lead to foreign body reactions, hypersensitivity, and biofilm production in some patients. Two of the most common stent materials are polylactide-co-glycolide (PLG), a bioabsorbable polymer used in the Propel family of stents (Intersect ENT, Menlo Park, CA), and Silastic.

Silicone and Silastic, widely used in medical devices such as cochlear implants, endotracheal, nasogastric, and laryngectomy tubes, have been reported to induce local fibrosis, foreign body reactions, and granuloma formation in some patients [12–13]. Sensitivities can be both immediate and delayed. Silastic is a silicone elastomer that is trademarked by the Dow Corning Corporation. All foreign bodies in the sinuses and airway, given sufficient time, will become colonized with microbes. Bacterial biofilms, which represent colonies of bacteria attached to a surface and to each other, are known to induce sinus mucosal inflammation. Perloff and Palmer found that 6/6 (100%) of Silastic stents removed in 1–4 weeks after FESS had bacterial biofilms on electron microscopy [14]. Nitinol sinus stents, which are comprised of nickel and titanium, can also act as a strong-antigenic compound leading to granulation tissue formation in the sinuses [10]. In such cases, stent removal is needed to allow for sinus mucosa normalization after FESS.

This antigenic response is not limited to non-dissolvable stents. Arguably, the most frequently used bioabsorbable stent in FESS, Propel, has been used in thousands of sinus cases yearly over the past 9 years. Contraindications to stent usage include to the active steroid ingredient, mometasone furoate, and patients with known hypersensitivities to the lactide, glycolide, or caprolactone copolymers that make up the implant [15]. Hypersensitivity reactions to corticosteroids are rare in the general population, estimated to be 0.3–0.5% [16]. Patients who elicit any history of steroid allergy or sensitivity to PLG sutures should not be considered candidates for steroid eluting implants in FESS.

Propel stents have been reported to cause local mucosal inflammation, granulation tissue, infection, and crusting necessitating early stent removal in a few cases [17]. In over 400 sinuses receiving the implant or a control implant (without steroid), the overall incidence of device-related adverse events was 1.5% due to recurrent sinusitis and nasal irritation [15]. The most recent Propel stent, Sinuva, meant for recurrent nasal polyps, can be left in the sinuses for up to 90 days. Complications requiring SINUVA removal in trials were low (<1%), suggesting that it is well-tolerated, but it is to be seen if repeated usage or long-term placement might lead to increased local reactions. When sinus symptoms persist despite evaluation and treatment for other inciting factors, stent-related hypersensitivity should be considered as a cause for post FESS inflammation or granulation tissue.

Stent Infection

Any foreign body, whether absorbable or nonabsorbable, carries the risk of infection when placed in the nasal cavity or sinuses. In some cases, these stents are left in place for months or permanently to prevent stenosis after FESS. Orlandi et al. reported his institution's experience with long-term frontal sinus stenting with Rains frontal sinus stents [18]. They reported that 1/9 (11%) of patients required stent removal due to chronic infection that could not be treated with culture-directed antibiotics. Another group reported chronic infection and granulation tissue due to a retained ethmoid stent that resolved after stent removal and culture-directed oral and topical antibiotics [11]. While rarely reported, absorbable stents have also been associated with infection before dissolving. The ADVANCE II study, which evaluates the use and safety of Propel bioabsorbable stents, reported that one of the 105 patients developed mucopurulence following removal of the control stent [17].

Toxic shock syndrome is a rare but devastating complication generally associated with nasal packing for epistaxis or after septorhinoplasty. Chadwell et al.

reported a rare but life-threatening complication of toxic shock syndrome related to frontal sinus stenting using Rains stents [9]. TSS is a rapidly progressive multiorgan system disease due to toxin-producing *Staphylococcus aureus*, first identified in 1978. The Center for Disease Control and Prevention (CDC) clinical criteria for TSS includes fever, rash, hypotension, and multisystem organ involvement [19]. On postoperative day 18, the patient presented to the emergency room with mental status change, fever, acute renal failure and a macular rash on the hands, feet, and trunk. Blood and sinus cultures were obtained both growing *Staphylococcus aureus*, and TSS toxin-1 was isolated confirming TSS syndrome. Surgeons should be aware of not only the risk of local stent infection, but also more serious complications such as sepsis or TSS.

Intracranial and Orbital Stent Placement

While uncommon, inadvertent placement of stents and spacers intracranially or in the orbit has occurred during FESS and can lead to significant morbidity. Our case highlights placement of a Rains stent intracranially after frontal sinus surgery, leading to a brain abscess and seizure. Other reports of skull base injury during ESS with stents have been associated with postoperative CSF rhinorrhea, mental status changes and pneumocephalus [6, 8]. These particular cases highlight important considerations when utilizing sinus stents: (1) confirmation of appropriate anatomic stent placement with direct visualization and (2) operative documentation of stent placement with subsequent timely removal of the stent.

Bone erosion has also been reported from prolonged stenting [8]. Studies have reported sinus stenting upward of 6 years without complication, and it is unknown what risk factors can lead to erosion of the skull base or orbit [8, 18]. Reeve et al. reported a case of prolonged frontal sinus stenting with a Rains stent leading to skull base erosion [8]. The stent was placed 8 years prior and was removed in the operating room without incident. Intact mucosa was seen around the stent with no visible CSF leak. As stent migration, dislocation, and malpositioning are all known risks of sinus stents, consideration should be given to periodic imaging after placement [8].

Tang et al. reported a fascinating case of a Propel spacer placed intracranially in a 70-year-old patient during FESS [6]. The patient had a very narrow frontal recess with a small anterior–posterior diameter, like our case, and the stent was placed intracranially. Presenting symptoms included mental status changes and headaches, while imaging demonstrated significant pneumocephalus. The patient had surgery to remove the spacer and the defect was reconstructed with a two-layer repair.

Stents are also commonly placed within the ethmoid region to prevent middle turbinate lateralization and adhesions. Though arguably easier to access compared to the frontal sinus, correct anatomic placement of stent material within the ethmoid sinus is still vital to avoid complications. Villari et al. reported a case of a drug-eluting stent placed through the lamina papyracea into the orbit leading to ocular pain, pressure and a fixed, dilated pupil [7]. The spacer was ultimately removed, but her pupil remained fixed and dilated at 2 months after surgery. This case highlights the need for direct visualization of stent placement. Orbital complaints after FESS should trigger concern for a complication necessitating a comprehensive ocular evaluation, endoscopy, and imaging with a low threshold for surgical re-exploration.

Lessons Learned

Stents have long been used to maintain sinus patency and to improve outcomes after FESS. Surgeons should bear in mind, that although stenting materials are selected and/or designed with biocompatibility in mind, they are not inert, and vigilance is required for potential immediate and delayed complications related to their use. While rare, foreign body reactions, infections, and complications due to incorrect stent placement have been reported and can be a significant source of persistent sinonasal symptoms and generalized morbidity.

References

1. Chin D, Snidvongs K, Kalish L, et al. The outside-in approach to the modified endoscopic Lothrop procedure. Laryngoscope. 2012;122(8):1661–9. https://doi.org/10.1002/lary.23319.
2. Yaniv D, Shlossberg L, Yaniv E. A prospective study on the safety and effectiveness of a composite sinus stent for use after endoscopic sinus surgery. Am J Rhinol Allergy. 2019;33(1):17–25. https://doi.org/10.1177/1945892418803101.
3. Chan C, Elmiyeh B, Woods C, et al. A randomized controlled trial of a middle meatal silastic stent for reducing adhesions and middle turbinate lateralization following endoscopic sinus surgery. Int Forum Allergy Rhinol. 2015;5(6):517–23. https://doi.org/10.1002/alr.21490.
4. Rains B III. Frontal sinus stenting. Otolaryngol Clin North Am. 2001;34(1):101–10. https://doi.org/10.1016/S0030-6665(05)70298-X.
5. Han J, Kern R. Topical therapies for management of chronic rhinosinusitis: steroid implants. Int Forum Allergy Rhinol. 2019;9:S22–6.
6. Tang D, Roxbury C, Sindwani R, et al. Multiple bioabsorbable corticosteroid-eluting stent placement with associated skull base injury. Laryngoscope. 2019;129:1494–6.
7. Villari C, Wojno T, DelGaudio J. Case report of orbital violation with placement of ethmoid drug-eluting stent. Int Forum Allergy Rhinol. 2012;2:89–92.
8. Reeve N, Ching H, Kim Y, et al. Possible skull base erosion after prolonged frontal sinus stenting. Ear Nose Throat J. 2019:145561319878951. https://doi.org/10.1177/0145561319878951.
9. Chadwell J, Gustafson L, Tami T. Toxic shock syndrome associated with frontal sinus stents. Otolaryngol Head Neck Surg. 2001;124(5):573–4.
10. Kounis N, Soufras G, Hahalis G. Stent hypersensitivity and infection in sinus cavities. Allergy Rhinol (Providence). 2013;4(3):e162–5. https://doi.org/10.2500/ar.2013.4.0071.
11. Sjogren P, Parker N, Boyer H. Retained drug-eluting stents and recalcitrant chronic rhinosinusitis: a case report. Allergy Rhinol (Providence). 2013;4(1):e45–8. https://doi.org/10.2500/ar.2013.4.0042.

12. O'Malley J, Burgess B, Galler D, et al. Foreign body response to silicone in cochlear implant electrodes in the human. Otol Neurotol. 2017;38(7):970–7. https://doi.org/10.1097/MAO.0000000000001454.
13. Rubio A, Ponvert C, Goulet O, et al. Allergic and nonallergic hypersensitivity reactions to silicone: a report of one case. Allergy. 2009;64(10):1555. https://doi.org/10.1111/j.1398-9995.2009.02086.
14. Perloff J, Palmer J. Evidence of bacterial biofilms on frontal recess stents in patients with chronic rhinosinusitis. Am J Rhinol. 2004;18(6):377–80.
15. Summary of safety and effectiveness data. PROPEL® Mini Sinus Implant. Intersect ENT. https://www.accessdata.fda.gov/cdrh_docs/pdf10/P100044S018b.pdf.
16. Vatti R, Ali F, Teuber S, et al. Hypersensitivity reactions to corticosteroids. Clin Rev Allergy Immunol. 2014;47(1):26–37. https://doi.org/10.1007/s12016-013-8365-z.
17. Marple B, Smith T, Han J, et al. ADVANCE II: a prospective, randomized study assessing safety and efficacy of bioabsorbable steroid-releasing sinus implants. Otolaryngol Head Neck Surg. 2012;146:1004–11.
18. Orlandi R, Knight J. Prolonged stenting of the frontal sinus. Laryngoscope. 2009;119(1):190–2.
19. Schmitz M, Roux X, Huttner B, et al. Streptococcal toxic shock syndrome in the intensive care unit. Ann Intensive Care. 2018;8(1):88.

Index

R. K. Chandra, K. C. Welch (eds.), *Lessons Learned from Rhinologic Procedure Complications*, https://doi.org/10.1007/978-3-030-75323-8

MIX
Papier aus verantwortungsvollen Quellen
Paper from responsible sources
FSC® C105338

If you have any concerns about our products,
you can contact us on
ProductSafety@springernature.com

In case Publisher is established outside the EU,
the EU authorized representative is:
Springer Nature Customer Service Center GmbH
Europaplatz 3, 69115 Heidelberg, Germany

Printed by Libri Plureos GmbH
in Hamburg, Germany